*"The fullness of joy is to behold
God in everything."*

Julian of Norwich

Grief to Gratitude

THE ART OF GRIEVING

Julie Kramer, M.P.H., M.A.

Grief to Gratitude

Copyright © 2021 by Julie Kramer, M.P.H., M.A.

All rights reserved. No part of this book may be reproduced or transmitted in any form or by any means without written permission of the author.

ISBN: 978-1-7365166-0-7

Table of Contents

Introduction 1
Chapter 1 Why I Wrote This Book 4
Chapter 2 My Story 8
Chapter 3 How to Work with Strands of Grief 13
Chapter 4 Six Benefits to Sharing Your Story 21
Chapter 5 An Open Heart Leads to Wisdom 28
Chapter 6 How Others Impact Your Grief Process 36
Chapter 7 The Soul's Perspective on Your Suffering 44
Chapter 8 What You Need to Know about Loss of Self 50
Chapter 9 How Inner Conflicts Perpetuate Grief 57
Chapter 10 Why a New Perspective Leads to Transformation 63
Chapter 11 The Art of Grieving 71
Resources 80
About The Author 81

Introduction

"Sorrow is better than laughter, for by sadness of countenance the heart is made glad."

— Ecclesiastes 7.3

This book is based on the ancient art of Spiritual Direction. Spiritual Direction is the process of uncovering the truth of things: the truth about your life, the truth about your needs and desires, the truth about your spiritual longings and the truth about your relationship with God. Spiritual Direction is the process of coming to terms with conflicts in your life. This includes conflicts about what you want, what others want and what you are being called toward.

The Spiritual Director is a spiritual friend or someone trained in the ways of the spiritual journey who guides you to connect more fully with yourself and with the Sacred. This process leads to understanding life's challenges from the point of view of your heart, your spirit, your soul and that of God. During the course of struggling with life's challenges — values and alliances can shift and pivot in a new direction.

As such, Spiritual Direction requires that you be emotionally and spiritually honest with yourself and open with God about your life circumstances. To the extent that you are emotionally and spiritually honest with yourself, you will open a window into the process of spiritual and emotional growth. This leads you to the truth of your heart's desires, your spirit's longings and your soul's calling.

In today's society it is typical to bring your struggles to a psychotherapist, but not to God. The approach presented in this book offers a structure for sharing your struggle with God. It provides a structure to find wisdom and new understanding that can arise out of loss and tragedy. *This approach emphasizes the transformative aspects of loss.*

It has been my experience that the combination of weeping, praying and seeking wisdom is transformative. I offer this process as the culmination of my lifelong struggle with sorrow and journey of recovery through grieving, praying, contemplation of scripture and seeking the wisdom from the Holy Spirit.

I have seen that a holistic approach, including ceremony, prayer, inner reflection and grieving, brings together the ingredients for transformation and growth. This is why each chapter is accompanied by a Candle-Lighting Prayer.

The word *God* in this book is meant to be all inclusive. Depending on your point of view and history, *God* may include Spirit, Beauty, Nature, Love, Higher Power, Ground of Being, Sacred Divine, or the Image of God within. Whatever the language and image of God is for you, I invite you to work with that. The main point is to relinquish your grief to God. To turn over and release of your sorrow, grief and anxiety is the foundation of this method.

Within these chapters, you are invited to experience loss from the perspective of creating beauty out of tragedy. You are invited to find a way to grieve that turns defeat, breakdown and destruction into innovation and new beginnings.

By looking at loss as the path to growth and emotional maturity, it becomes a completely different experience. Without loss, there is no growth. In loss, something leaves to make room for something else. Often the "something else" turns out to be invaluable: It makes life richer, deeper and more worthwhile. *There is an art to grieving*, just as there is an art to cooking, communicating or gardening. It is a process of creation. It is life-giving. If you can just bear the pain and endure through it to new understanding, you will grow into a new person.

What I have also discovered is when grief becomes stuck in emotional pitfalls (such as anger, fear, despair and numbness), it is simply from a lack of understanding about the *art* of the process.

The *Art of Grieving* includes a number of elements: feeling your feelings, sorting out your feelings, contemplating the pros and cons, seeing the beauty in the suffering and finally getting to that bittersweet place where you are both sad and happy at the same time. There, you hold both the pain of the loss and the blessing of what came afterward all in your heart at one time. In other words, it's that paradoxical place where two opposites co-exist.

This approach works with story (mind) feelings (heart), spirit (sacred ceremony) so that all aspects of Self are engaged in the process. The ongoing "conversation" between the different aspects of Self keeps the process engaging.

This approach is based on recognition of the Sacred as the ground of all being and the forum through which difficulties may be resolved and understood — creating new perspectives, new wisdom and new blessings. By way of the Sacred, you can discover that there is blessing and wisdom in your suffering.

The power of this process is that it allows you notice that you are in a new state of mind, which you would not have reached without experiencing the loss. It is important to celebrate the inspiration, wisdom and enrichment of where you arrived *simultaneously* to grieving the loss. The combination of both activities at once creates a powerful state change.

This process is partly the work of the heart, partly the work of the mind and partly the work of the spirit. Your work is to dwell on and contemplate the loss while seeking broader and deeper emotional meaning in order to finally celebrate the illumination that came out of the loss. This is a deliberate seeking resulting in a significant and eloquent shift in perception. This leads to emotional intelligence and wisdom.

It is my intention that through this book you will learn how to *go through grief fast and thoroughly* while mining the wisdom. That way, you will end up in a new place of gratitude and joy. You will arrive at a place of immense love — love for yourself, love for others, love for God and love for life's possibilities.

Chapter 1
Why I Wrote This Book

Many have argued that Western civilization is built around the Denial of Death (and grief) and follows the Way of the Mind over the Way of the Heart. After eight years of working in the San Francisco Bay Area as a hospital and hospice chaplain, I would have to agree with this assertion.

During the economic downturn in 2000, I decided to try out a new career. I had heard about the work of hospice chaplains during my time at seminary, and became curious because this spiritual work is so different from that of a minister or pastor. Chaplains spend most of their time in pastoral care, working directly with people in crisis (family conflicts, estrangement, homelessness, disagreements, unfulfilled longings) who are experiencing a wide range of feelings (regret, doubt, fear, anxiety, anger, sorrow, depression). Part of a chaplain's job is to give witness to these feelings and reflect support and encouragement. I soon learned that people move quickly from one feeling to the next and keeping up was part of my job.

Having come from the corporate world, the jump to being a chaplain was like night and day—a jarring transition that forced me to make big changes. Suddenly experiencing many unexpected situations, I had to move from the objective to the subjective, from theoretical to immediate, from implementing prepackaged standardized solutions to inventing my own solution on the spot. Through it all, I discovered a love for this work and the creativity it required. It felt much more like "real work."

After sharing time with thousands of people on the edge of death—or going thru major life crises—I discovered that grief was usually the missing ingredient for a safe journey through crisis and onto a positive resolution. Because of this, it is not surprising that these people were stuck in bitter debates about what to do and how to proceed, including how to deal with caregiving choices, legal issues and financial matters at the end of life. I found that most people were approaching their trials from a point of view that focused on the mind and bypassed the realm of the heart, spirit and soul.

In almost every instance a sister or brother, husband or wife, grandparents or grandchildren were locked in disagreements at the bedside of someone who was either dying, in crisis or undergoing a great loss.

As a new chaplain, I was faced with either adding value to the situation—or leaving the room. The reason for this, is that people dealing with a grave crisis, when confronted with a stranger, demand that the stranger (chaplain or not) add value to their situation. In order to stay in the room, I had to reengineer the dynamics. My job as a chaplain, as opposed to just being an annoying stranger, was to find ways to add value for these people who were in anger, grief, fear and sometimes bitterness.

My role was to help people connect with the Divine, to lean on it, and to get help and inspiration during a stressful time. But, I found that there were many obstacles to fulfilling my role as a chaplain. One obstacle was that people gathered around a bedside may be of different faiths. Another is that people may have stopped praying—stopped listening to the divine—because they had become numb and were unable to pray any longer. Still another obstacle is that hospitals are dominated by an informational, fact-based way of thinking and communicating. This scenario does not honor the value of emotions.

My job was figuring out how to add value to these situations.

The primary challenge was that people were polarized and unable to make choices. They were often amplifying divisions, getting more and more opinionated, judgmental, and angry with one another. And oftentimes appealing to reason only made the problem worse. The solution lay in moving the conversation from their minds to their hearts, getting them to shift towards an emotional reality where reconciliation was possible.

The question was how to shift the conversation from the realm of the mind (with all of the associated judgments, opinions and fears) to the realm of the heart. This is a problem—getting stuck in the intellectual way of looking at things—that I was familiar with.

My personal solution eventually became praying, having found that it opens the heart. Since this worked for me personally it became what I brought to the people gathered around those beds, using prayer to get people back in touch with their feelings. Some of these prayers are offered in this book to help you get unstuck.

I discovered that talking helps get in touch with the heart's way of knowing—as does grief. Eventually, I came to invite people to speak about their sorrow, fear, worries, and to share their tears, making room for weeping and welcoming the grief as people opened up more and more.

This led to creating a structured set of open-ended questions, inquiries and questions:

- What has this person given you?
- What have you given them?
- What was the contribution of this person's life to the world?
- What do you want to thank them for?
- What do you want forgiveness for?
- What do you forgive them for?

By letting people know that their grief was welcome—and even essential—to the process, they came to understand that they had permission to weep. The "intellectuals" in the group given stern warnings not to interrupt the grief. Such ground rules made these moments successful, which inspired me to create ceremonies that brought it all together: music, prayers and people's words into a single holistic event.

And it worked! They moved into their hearts. The result was a powerful, deep and authentic experience. Combining inquiry, weeping, prayer and music changed the dynamic completely. Miracles happened. Things began to move. This is when I realized that grief was the glue that brought it all together and saw that this was the missing piece in the process.

After nine years working as a chaplain and grief counselor, it became clear how entrenched we are in **not** grieving. This book is meant to share a method that works, one which promotes the idea that grief is healing, and to generate a revival in the art of grieving. **We all need to grieve**. It's an argument for the value of grieving.

The stories in this book are meant to inspire you to try it yourself and discover the miracles that come from grieving. These stories are only a tiny fraction of what my work allowed me to bear witness to, the hundreds of miracles where lives were restored with new meaning, new focus and new direction. There is an *Art to Grieving* which, once learned, is very energizing.

Based on working with approximately 10,000 people, it has been my experience that when people are guided through the *Art of Grieving*, they acquire wisdom, experience a transformation and come to create a well-lived life.

The results of my system were so fantastic that I wanted to document its methodology. It is a system that can be used to heal, pivot, renew and find depth and hope and faith.

First self-published with a CD in 2007 as *Grief to Gratitude*, I used it with clients who were trapped in their grief. It became a tool to argue my case to them: that there was a way to permanently process and release their grief.

Because the results were so profound, I began to wonder if it could be expanded into more general griefwork as a way to help heal people with non-life-threatening problems. To test this idea out, I offered a half-day workshop with ten people. After four hours, this group experienced a dramatic shift from sorrow to love. At the end of the workshop we arrived at a place of wonder and awe and found that the method worked.

My initial goal was learning if the method would work—meaning did it move the people out of their heads and into their hearts, readying them to open themselves to self-examination and self-forgiveness? Did they release old hurts and welcome Divine wisdom? Did they get an inkling of their soul's desires? And they did all of this. But they did more.

The great surprise was that everyone was healed and three-to-six months later almost everyone in the workshop got in touch to tell me so. I was astonished. This was more than I had expected. That experience led to this book.

There is a prevailing myth that grief is with you forever, that there is nothing you can do about it. This is not true. There is a way. This book provides a system with a roadmap which I invite you to follow.

Chapter 2
My Story

I was raised by a working-class family passionate about labor union organizing and creating better working conditions for blue-collar workers. My family's circle included artists, writers and union activists who formed an enclave of alternative thinkers, including a wide range of people like a Pulitzer Prize winner, a prominent attorney, and a respected labor union leader (as well as some fanatics, sociopaths, psychotics and narcissists). Living this way—on the fringe of society as an outcast from the mainstream—led to the ability to cope in two different worlds, speak two different languages and see life from two different perspectives. I was reminded of this daily.

By the age of 12, I had developed a passionate desire to become a regular person—like I thought everyone else was—with a respectable career. But the challenge was my feeling of being rejected, year after year, by mainstream people. This launched me on my journey.

I struggled to be accepted, up to and including graduate school. Due to continuous rejection, I became sensitive to people's attitudes, beliefs and feelings, and spent most of my free time learning how to "fit in." This led to becoming a lifelong learner and seeker who read every self-help book remotely connected to my struggles.

Struggle to Overcome

Depression was a constant aspect of my life for about 25 years while I sought answers. I explored over 250 personal growth methodologies including coaching, therapy, communication programs, nonviolent communication, yoga, meditation, dance therapy, Al-Anon, healing programs, spiritual direction, co-active listening, voice dialogue, psychotherapy, prayer, and journal writing.

Struggle to Find My Purpose

Hired out of graduate school by a prestigious consulting firm to develop long-range plans for large hospitals, I went on to hold several excellent positions in Chicago, including director of planning for a large facility.

Although each job was very sexy and exciting—throwing me into the midst of big corporate deals, multimillion-dollar grant applications, and brainstorming on cutting-edge issues—something was not quite right.

Restless, I left this series of jobs in Chicago while working to improve my communication skills to become more assertive, a better negotiator and better able to frame issues to persuade and educate people with oppositional views. Assessing the character and motivation of people—to draw out the needs of others, to not offend and to advance to ideas—was key. I learned the rules of the corporate game, how to identify political agendas, personalities, motivations and character traits and to read between the lines to better understand what people were really saying. Dealing with self-centered, aggressive, manipulative, dishonest and ruthless people was part of the deal. Very idealistic, I thought framing issues correctly would make people go with my agenda, not realizing that other issues— personality traits, values, styles, norms and agendas—were at play. Part of the toolbox for surviving in the corporate world included knowing how to deal with a wide range of people and how the corporate political game worked. Burnt out, I left Chicago after trying to remake myself into someone other than who I really was.

This was the **first turning point**, which included a year off and falling into a depression. Leaving my entire career behind—built on an MBA in Medical Care Administration and Planning—felt like a divorce. I eventually moved back to San Francisco and into a new career with an executive search firm, work that took me inside of the minds of corporate executives. Countless interviews with CEOs at Fortune 500 companies led to understanding their worldview, including the realization that executives have all kinds of problems. Frequently, there are vision, mission and value conflicts within their board of directors, executive team and between the CEO and the CFO (or all of the above). At the executive level, there may also be conflicts between senior Vice Presidents and the C-suite over vision, mission and goals.

Simultaneously, I was struggling with my family of origin, feeling misunderstood and without the ability to make any headway. This was a significant blow. There was a great deal of anguish in my life; eventually, I enrolled in the seminary, looking for emotional and spiritual support. I took up the study of values and value conflicts. **This was the second turning point.**

By the end of my program, (MA Arts and Values), I began to understand that people may have very different values; and that you have to accept these differences before deciding how to deal with them. What can you live with? And when do you need to make a stand or articulate an alternative point of view?

Frankly, this is one of the most important things we learn in life. It became clear that my family of origin and I had many fundamental conflicts about core values.

In 1990, I enrolled in a master's program in Systematic Theology at the Graduate Theological Union, studying theology, spirituality, worship and Christian history. I conducted worship services, entered into spiritual direction and experienced the power of prayer to could change beliefs, circumstances, feelings and outcomes. This discovery of prayer was very powerful and it began my healing.

Even so, I still felt the pull of my mainstream career and in 1995 I left the seminary to work for a number of leading-edge start-ups like Netscape, Organic Online, LookSmart, E*Trade and a Venture Capital Search firm. Despite the initial excitement of such work, the feeling that I was not really serving people—or working with depth—began to set-in. Sleepless nights while restlessly searching for something more led to the realization that this was not my calling. I had landed a terrific job with an executive search firm but left it in 2000 to become trained as a chaplain.

I spent a month trying out chaplain work, including meeting a 90-year old in a nursing home who brought me to a turning point. She came alive during our time together, which was thrilling, and my **third turning point**. A glimmer of my true calling had become clear.

But there were obstacles ahead.

Obstacles

I decided to try chaplain work for a year and, if I didn't like it, to go back to corporate work. But first, I had to negotiate with my inner critic who was certain that this path would drain my retirement savings while paying too little day-to-day. That it was, rationally speaking, an unsafe career path, was very true. There were few jobs for chaplains, they were usually part-time, and the pay was about a fourth of my corporate income. Bargaining with parts of myself that were in powerful conflict commenced as my inner critic was strongly opposed to the idea. But, rising to the occasion, my inner artist took charge and a huge battle ensued. After a year of chaplain work—during which I witnessed the people I served moving from confusion to clarity, from despair to hope, and from grief to joy—my supervisor told me I had a gift for the work.

Gradually gaining confidence, I began to realize that this was my true calling. Being a chaplain, meant working with people at deeper levels which brought me alive again. The work also involved witnessing miracles.

While assisting people to find their passion for life, to reconcile with their families and circumstances, and connect with the divine, I also enrolled in

Coach Training Program and became a life coach. I began to blend tools from Life Coaching with the tools of Spiritual Direction.

Trained at both the UCSF Medical Center and the Mercy Center for Spiritual Direction, over the next eight years I served people going through life-threatening challenges, helping them understand their life in relationship to God and talking about how they could move forward into the next stage of faith. Beauty and spirit worked together and prayer called forth new realities. People struggled with the questions like: "What does it mean to have had a well-lived life?" and "What is Love?" and "What does a life that values Love look like?" Wrestling with these same questions while listening to hundreds of people informs my work as a spiritual director and gives me a foundation for dealing with a very broad range of religious and spiritual issues.

As a chaplain and spiritual director, I had to go into the emptiness, let go of all I had learned and find new ways of being. This meant embracing deep listening, grief counseling and the exploration of gratitude forgiveness.

Creating prayer ceremonies to celebrate life and death, love and loss, and lifetime milestones with families taught me how prayer, ceremony, release, celebration and acknowledgment can bring people out of grief or resentment and back into love.

The Method

My many struggles in life, and my experience as a chaplain, led to the creation of my **own method**. This is based on training in Spiritual Direction, Value Conflicts and Life Coaching. This method evolved from working with 10,000 people from all walks of life, of various ages and religious orientations, all of whom had a wide range of problems. Learning to listen deeply, understand the problem and choose which tool to use was a huge part of the work.

It has been my experience that, during times of transition, people may shut down due to conflict between perspectives. The method I developed works with these variable perspectives.

The three primary elements of my method are:

- A way to process grief, fear, anger and loss
- A way to pivot, get unstuck and move to new perspectives
- A way to authentically reconnect to the divine

This approach enables people to get unstuck and pivot quickly, to negotiate deeply buried inner conflicts and focus on a bigger vision that emanates from, and with, and through the divine.

A few examples of such inner conflicts include:
- Conflicts between the heart and mind
- Conflicts between the creative and the practical
- Conflicts between the idealist and the realist.

For example, if a person's perspective is based on analytical and methodical thinking, they may perceive their options using only linear thinking, logic and facts. Or if the person tends to be more creative—with thinking based on artistic, intuitive, rhythmic, and holistic approaches—they may come up with an entirely different set of options.

My method helps a person become consciously aware of such differing perspectives, pulling them into owning these different perspectives and the ability to wrestle with them. This includes mediation to broaden horizons and understand aspects of both sides while releasing what is out of date or no longer true. This liberates the person to flow with reality and reengage with their values, their soul's calling and their life's purpose.

While applying this system, I witnessed miraculous healings, reconciliations and transformations.

What distinguishes my coaching method from the approach of others is that we dive to the depths of your heart, soul and spirit to find your true purpose and life mission. We connect to the divine for wisdom and grace while processing the grief of your losses. It is an original system for getting unstuck and reconnecting to your core values—and your best path in life.

For the past 18 years I have built, expanded and refined my processes to recover from wounds, challenges and divisions. This includes coaching people in all stages of life, with diverse and various religious affiliations, levels of spirituality and values to resolve their issues and move to a place of peace and harmony.

My mission today is to work with people to help them discover where they want to go and how to break through barriers to find new perspectives, visions and goals. I coach a wide range of people in a wide range of transitional situations. If you would like to explore working with me, I invite you to visit my website:

www.kramercoaching.com

You may contact me at julie@kramercoaching.com.

Chapter 3
How to Work with Strands of Grief

"The problem is ... basically: how to remain whole in the midst of the distractions of life; how to remain balanced, no matter what centrifugal forces tend to pull us off center; how to remain strong, no matter what shocks come in at the periphery and tend to crack the hub of the wheel."

— Anne Morrow Lindbergh

Grief is like a ball of string. You may think you are only grieving about one event or circumstance, but that string (or strand) of grief is connected to something else — and that "something else" is connected to many more things. As it all unravels it becomes overwhelming, which begets hopelessness. And once you become hopeless, fears run rampant. You may be afraid of becoming "shut down" or emotionally paralyzed by the sheer magnitude of the grief being experienced. At that point, it's likely your "protective side" will put the brakes on the whole grieving process because it feels too dangerous.

That "Protector" is right; it is dangerous to become submerged in sorrow. The trick to grieving is to engage and experience the grief *without becoming hopeless*.

One effective way to grieve from a safe and protected place is to "wall off" parts while you focus exclusively on a particular subset of despair or discomfort. That way, you can take one niche of grief at a time and work through it.

The following exercise will take 10-15 minutes and is designed to help you see the breadth and magnitude of the loss or transition you're going through ... without getting "stuck" in it. Afterward, you'll have a clear overview of your grief. But it's essential that you don't become bogged down by this experience. Be aware of how you're feeling, and if you find yourself getting "caught up" in your sorrow, take a break. Go for a walk or call a friend. Continue when you feel the time is right.

The View From 10,000 Miles

Start by briefly reviewing the many facets and layers of your grief. Now, look at it from "the 10,000-mile perspective." Imagine you are up in the cosmos looking down at yourself.

You have the advantage of millions of perspectives from your vantage point. Now, speed through your situation. Do a fast review of the events leading up to this point in your life.

You might go back one year, three years or even 10 years, but do not dwell long on any one event.

Now that you've reviewed the chronology, do a quick review of all the people involved in your current sorrow. Again, don't dwell on any one person. Just list them all in your mind.

Having examined the individuals involved, next review *your actions* leading up to and during this time of sorrow.

Now you have the big panorama. You have the series of events, the variety of people, the things they said and you said and the losses involved. The reason for starting here is to create a clear picture of the landscape you are going to be dealing with throughout this book, and to choose which part of the landscape you want to begin with. By identifying all the parts of the big picture, you can give yourself permission to *start somewhere* and just let the rest go until a later time.

It's a way to organize the journey.

It's also a way to step back from all that's happened and acknowledge its size and scope. As you see the magnitude of your loss and your psyche acknowledges it, you have a chance to broaden your perspective and move forward emotionally. That is to say, your heart can feel the enormity and the depth of those sorrowful events in a new way — a way that honors what happened and changes your outlook.

This program is organized in a specific way that allows you to take one strand of grief at a time and work it through the entire book, from beginning to end. Then afterward, you can take the second strand of grief and work it through the entire book from beginning to end, and so on. This method mitigates against being overcome by sorrow. In some circles, this is called "chunking it down." The value of taking one strand at a time is in the way it lets you focus on that one piece of your experience long enough to actually process it into a new energy. And then it's gone, and you can start with the next strand.

At this point, it's time to list all the strands of grief you identified in the previous exercise. You can list them by events, people, actions or circumstances. And your list could be as short as five or 10 things, or as long as 20 or 30 things.

If your list is longer than 30 items, then consolidate the items into categories. Write them down in the lined space provided.

Reflect on the stands of grief with which you are dealing. Strands of grief are the components of your sorrow coming from different foundations. For example, an immediate loss may be connected to another loss in the past. So these are two different strands. Or your loss may have different parts to it such as conflicts that came up with friends and family over the loss, conflicts that came up within yourself over your own values, or conflicts with institutions (hospitals, corporations or employers). Other conflicts may include disappointment around legal requirements, contractual agreements, settlements or the process through which you had to go.

The reason for clarifying the strands of your sorrow is so that you can see which one carries more weight, which one is more important to you right now and which one is within closest proximity to your heart.

The strands of grief are all connected. If you have lost a loved one, you have grief. But this loss may remind you of another loss earlier in your life, and you may end up grieving both losses at once. In a similar way, if you have lost your job, you may experience the related grief of a firing from another job … or being passed over for a promotion … or the time you had to take off from work to tend to other matters … or the sacrifices you made in your career for the sake of your family. It is this *interconnectivity of grief* that makes it so useful to focus on one isolated strand at a time, all the way from beginning to end.

A woman was in the process divorcing her husband and was utterly despondent. She was in despair about the loss of her marriage, but it also brought up her relationship with her father. He had been an alcoholic and absentee parent for much of her childhood. Those memories conjured thoughts of her first husband, also an alcoholic, who died. She had so many linked strands of grief that it was overwhelming. In fact, her experience was so overwhelming she was tempted to stuff it all down and forget about it. But as we focused on one strand of grief at a time, it was possible to work through it all.

Scripture Reading

The Scripture Reading in each chapter was selected to help you to see the universality of grief and to see how loss is part of the human condition. You are invited to read the following scripture aloud. Let yourself be comforted knowing that this is part of your humanity — that by embracing your grief, you are actually saying "yes" to life:

"For my life is spent with sorrow, and my years with sighing; my strength fails because of my misery, bones waste away."

— Psalm 31:10

Contemplation

Because the process of contemplation eventually leads to letting go of grief, it is helpful to set the context for grieving in a way that invites curiosity. A context of curiosity engages you to inquire further into the nature of your grief. And by looking deeper into your grief, you begin to unravel it, clarify it and understand it. You are invited on this journey as you consider the following questions:

1. Reflect on the strands of your loss.
2. List the strands of your loss on the next page. Examples include:
   - Loss of a loved one
   - Loss of income or residence
   - Loss of future plans
   - Related losses and conflicts
   - Loss of friendship from a conflict
   - Disappointment over settlements or outcomes
   - Disillusionment with institutions
   - Regret, guilt or shame
3. What is the most important strand of your loss today? What tugs at your heart the most?
4. What is beyond your focus at this time?
5. What does not belong to you that you can release?

List the strands of loss and grief you are now holding:

_____
_____
_____
_____
_____
_____
_____
_____
_____
_____
_____
_____
_____
_____
_____
_____
_____
_____
_____
_____
_____

Please continue to the next page …

After you have listed all the strands, listen to your heart and what it tells you is the most important strand of grief today. "Most important" means the strand that tugs at your heartstrings the most. Which strand can you not seem to get out of your memory bank? Which strand do you find yourself thinking about all the time? This is the strand to focus on throughout the rest of the book. After you complete the entire book, take the next strand and work that through each chapter, and so on.

Now spend a minute or two reflecting on each strand of grief. Which strands are constantly tugging at you for attention? Which strands are beyond your focus at this time? Which strands belong to other people and are not your concern?

Candle-Lighting Prayer for Release

The following prayer has been developed to enable you to release each strand of grief and offer it to God for keeping. The idea behind this prayer is to introduce the breadth and the depth of your suffering to God by naming each strand of your loss. As you present each strand of loss to God, keep the intention in your heart that *"God will provide me with direction, wisdom and nurturing for this process."* Also, hold faith that in releasing these strands of grief, there is something to be learned and gained and known from the suffering you've experienced.

This is an overview of the process you'll go through later with your chosen strand of grief. But right now, as a way of beginning, you can offer each strand to God today. This will give you a sense of the process you'll experience much deeper when working with your individual strands of grief in Chapters 2-9. This prayer is not meant as a substitute for that deeper process yet to come; it is merely the beginning of your process of working through grief to wisdom and gratitude.

During the prayer, you will look over the strands of grief you listed on the worksheet. You will focus on each strand one-by-one and light a candle for that strand of sorrow as you review the scope of it in your heart. At the end, you will recite the following words aloud and ask for God to release your sorrows from your heart and spirit. You will ask for Spirit to take these sorrows from your heart and replace them with wisdom.

Recite these words aloud:

Creative Source of All Being
      Bring my spirit into Your presence
Eternal Spirit of the Universe
      Align my hopes with Yours
Giver of Love
      Open my heart to love
Giver of All Good and Perfect Gifts
      Prepare me to receive
Searcher of Hearts
      Illuminate my sorrows
Shining Glory
      Lift me to Your glory
Source of All True Joy
      Remind me again of joy
Source of Blessing
      Bring forth Your blessing
Source of Creation
      I honor You as the source of all
Source of Good
      I honor the true and the good
Source of Life
      Remind me that You are the source of life and death
Source of Peace
      Prepare me to receive Your peace
Source of Mercy
      I ask for Your mercy
Source of Strength
      Let me lean on You for courage
Source of Truth
      Show me the truth in the midst of this loss

Sovereign God

I present to You my brokenness, anger and disappointment.
I present to You my regret, trauma and suffering.
I present to You my grief and sorrow.

I come before You today to honor all that You are
To open myself to all these aspects of Your being
To witness Your power and glory
To be transformed by Your love and grace.

Now present the first strand (verbally and by name) to God as you light a candle for that strand. Ask the Divine to receive this strand of sorrow on your behalf and share with you some wisdom from this loss. Allow yourself enough time to sit with the sorrow and imagine God receiving it from you, and to imagine hearing what God might say about this loss ... When you are finished, continue with the rest of the prayer by reciting these words:

God, shepherd me through this journey.
God, protect me from hopelessness.
God, hold my sorrow with wisdom.
God, transform each strand of this loss into energy and hope.

I dedicate this time to this end in the name of God.

Now sit for a few minutes in silence to contemplate what you have just done. Consider the magnitude of the losses. Consider the complexities. Consider the time period over which this has occurred.

Repeat this prayer for each strand of your grief. Keep in mind that as you move on to the next chapter, you will only be focusing on the first strand of your grief. Work that strand through all the chapters before repeating the process with the next strand.

Chapter 4
Six Benefits to Sharing Your Story

"We have no reason to mistrust our world, for it is not against us. Has it terrors, they are our terrors; has it abysses, those abysses belong to us; are dangers at hand, we must try to love them ... Perhaps everything terrible is in its deepest being something helpless that wants help from us."

— Rainer Maria Rilke

Sharing your story is a key part of the grieving process because it honors the loss, the learning and the wisdom gained from going through the experience. Your story can shine light on the rich tapestry of your memories and link you to your legacy, your history and your future. This can be passed on to others going through similar losses.

The first benefit from sharing your story, is that it brings emotional depth and gives your life a fuller, richer context. The process of sharing is mentally stimulating, lowers stress and relieves elements of depression.

The second benefit from recounting the story of your loss is that it creates a truthful record that lays the groundwork for recovery. This is therapeutic because it helps you to reach closure sooner about significant losses.

The third benefit of telling the story of all that you went through, is that it is a way of tapping into the wisdom of your experience. As you tell your story, you will look at the path taken and the wisdom gained along the way.

The fourth benefit of telling your story, is that it brings clarity to who you are, what your purpose is and what values you hold. In this way, telling your story has the power to bring you out of your sorrow. Your story may also introduce parts of you that have been suppressed. You may find new strengths and begin to trust yourself, trust what you believe and trust who you are ... and *why* you are that person.

The fifth benefit of telling your story, is that you document your unique journey — with its challenges, decisions and losses. All that you went through becomes a valuable resource for yourself, friends, family and others you meet who are on the same journey.

This documentation can build expertise for you to use later in building your legacy and doing volunteer work or caregiving work.

The sixth benefit of sharing what's happened is that it uncovers your "values in action." By focusing on how you reacted to stress, challenge and adversity, you gain clarity on what you did and what happened. If you made a mistake, reflection on how this made you feel lets you move back into a place of integrity. Reviewing the story of events, clarifies your values, your history and your legacy.

To summarize, the six benefits from sharing your story include: emotional depth, closure, wisdom, clarity of purpose, your legacy and you values.

Storytelling is an emotional experience, and when you share your stories with others it can create intimacy, bonding and a strong sense of connection. If there are family or friends involved in your loss, you may want to invite them to join you in telling the story of what happened. This sets up an environment where the emotional experience can be shared and people can get to know each other better. Family and friends who share their stories with one another strengthen the connections between them. This, in turn, creates a more supportive community of support for you.

I invite you to begin now to fully share your story — either aloud or to a friend or family member. One way to begin is to write it down in a journal. Another way is to call up a friend and ask that person to listen to your story. Otherwise, you might want to take a walk in nature with a tape recorder and tell your story aloud while you walk.

To encourage you to get started, here is an account of someone whose despair was significantly diminished by telling her story of loss:

In my work as a hospital chaplain, I met a woman who had been bedridden for about two years. Her initial illness was lupus, which was later compounded with multiple infections, a broken hip and then a cancerous tumor. As she recounted the story of the past few years of her life, I began to understand that she had been brooding over the betrayal of trust by her family. While she was bedridden, she spent a good deal of time remembering the hurtful things that had been said to her and about her — and the misrepresentation of truth about her motives and goals.

The more she thought about this the sicker she became.

I learned that her family had lied to her, put her life at risk and taken advantage of her. Over several weeks, she told me her story over and over.

Each time, I asked her new questions, such as:

- "What do you make of this?"
- "What have you lost?"
- "What does this say about your values?"
- "Who are you?"

The process of telling her story brought meaning and value to her life journey. It gave her a context for her distress.

It created emotional depth. In the end, telling the story of her losses gave her a sense of appreciation for her courage and honor in the face of adversity.

She began to acquire a new respect for, and commitment to, her values. By the fifth telling of her story, she realized that her values were significantly different than the values of her family. She began to realize the impossibility of sustaining an intimate connection with people who hold opposing values. She became clear on the worth of her life and her desire to continue living. She created a truthful record of all that she had gone through and began to appreciate her strengths.

Scripture Reading

You are invited to read the following scripture aloud:

"Choose sorrow over laughter because a sad face may hide a happy heart. A sensible person mourns but fools always laugh."

— Ecc 7:3

Contemplation

In Chapter 1, you selected the "most important" strand of your grief to work on. Take a few minutes to focus on your feelings related to this strand. Take time to sit still and reflect on the experience. You can do this by speaking aloud, writing down your feelings or listening to contemplative music. The goal is to listen to what your heart is telling you. Listening involves clearing out the *thoughts* from your mind so you can *feel* the pain from the experience. Keep your focus on your feelings rather than shifting it back to your thoughts, judgments or opinions.

Now that you have selected your first strand of grief, take some time to contemplate the following questions from your heart's perspective. Write down your answers in the space provided:

1. What key events are related to this strand of grief?
2. What was the history of events?
3. What circumstances arose to complicate matters?
4. What is the meaning of these events for you?
5. What effect did this have on you?
6. What was out of your control that you can let go of now?
7. What are your feelings and needs now?

Notice your heart's calling from this experience.

These questions are designed to help you review your story and all the aspects of it, specific to this first strand of grief. While it's easy to get off on a tangent, try to be disciplined and focused on staying with this one strand. For example, if your loved one died *and* someone behaved poorly toward you — but your first strand is focused on the actual death of your loved one — don't focus on what that someone else did. The impact of others' behavior will be covered a later chapter.

If you realize now that your thoughts or feelings strayed from your first strand onto tangential matters, take a moment to revisit the questions above.

There may have been a series of situations, circumstances and events that when all combined created traumatic upset. Note the events in sequential order and write them down. Notice how much time has passed from beginning to end. Now that you have noticed the magnitude of the loss situation, choose one event (with a specific day and time) to work on processing. Within that specific day and time, select a specific event that you would like to release … Now notice the magnitude of what you have gone through.

List the traumatic events in sequential order and write them down here:

_____
_____
_____
_____
_____
_____
_____
_____
_____
_____
_____
_____
_____
_____
_____
_____
_____
_____
_____

Please continue to the next page ...

Candle-Lighting Prayer

This program encourages you to explore your relationship with God and to draw closer to God by way of contemplation and prayer. Both are important to put your loss into perspective. Contemplation and prayer help you to see the magnitude of your loss and to honor your endurance for living through such a life-changing experience. Contemplation and prayer invite you into the depth of your sorrow. Contemplation offers you a way to acknowledge what you went through and to step back to see that it was a big deal. Prayer gives you a way to remember that God is there for you, which you may sometimes forget. Prayer makes it easier to forgive yourself for being angry or sad. And prayer helps you hold your heart open when you have lost something or someone you care about deeply.

Through prayer, you find the light in the dark and the blessing in the loss. As you discover the blessing, you are able to complete your grieving and understand that you have done a great work because you've preserved the integrity of your heart.

Without prayer, there is a danger of becoming involved in judgment, anger and blame. This can lead to becoming too angry and losing your heart's openness to love and life. It's a terrible thing to close your heart because of a loss, and prayers invite you ask God for reconnection with Self, with your spirit and with your hopes and dreams. Prayer creates a pathway to healing your heart's wounds and leads you back to love again. Prayer helps your spirit let go of things that are no longer useful. Prayer gives you a way to move with Spirit into intuition.

Consider your grief from this perspective as you say the following Candle-Lighting Prayer aloud:

Welcome Sacred Spirit,
Welcome Abundant Grace
You who are gracious and just
You who live in truth
Whose ways are loving
Who blesses and loves
Those who open their hearts.

Thanks for Your wisdom and truth
Thanks for Your vast majesty
Thanks for the breadth of Your stride.

I confess this unbearable loss
Which brought forth angst and bitterness
Which brought forth resentments and shame
Which brought forth anger and fury.

I confess my broken heart
With its longings, disappointments, dreads
Fears, agitations, irritations,
Loneliness, sorrow, helplessness,
Exhaustions and embarrassments.

I confess pain and discomfort
From this loss of routine,
Loss of perspective
Loss of balance
Loss of steady passion.

Gracious God, I give to You this loss *(Light a candle.)*
And all the ruminations of my heart
That came out of this loss.
I give over this tempest of feelings
Into Your care and friendship.

Sacred God, One who transforms sorrow into wisdom
Receive these sorrows from me to You *(Light a candle.)*
Protect me and free me
Renew me and fill me.

Precious Loving God,
Please affirm my worth, value and honor.
Please affirm my life and humanity.
I light this candle to present this request. *(Light a candle.)*
Thank you for answers to these prayers.

Chapter 5
An Open Heart Leads to Wisdom

"Pain comes from experiencing life just as it is; with no trimmings. We can even call this direct experiencing joy. But when we try to run away and escape from our experience of pain, we suffer. Freedom is the willingness to risk being vulnerable to life."
— Charlotte Joko Beck

For centuries, the heart has been considered the source of emotion, courage and wisdom. The Institute of HeartMath in Santa Cruz, Calif., has been exploring the physiological mechanisms by which the heart communicates with the brain and influences information processing, perceptions, emotions and health. The Institute has worked on questions of the heart and studied how stressful emotional states affect the autonomic nervous system, the hormonal and immune systems, the heart and the brain. After 20 years of work, this research and training organization has scientifically proved that heart rate variability and heart rhythms are the most important factors for inner emotional states. They have found that negative emotions lead to increased disorder in the heart and the nervous system and this adversely affects the rest of the body. They have proved that positive emotions create increased harmony in heart rhythms and improve the nervous system.

The HeartMath research shows that the rhythm of the heart affects:

- mental clarity
- creativity
- emotional balance
- pain reduction
- respiration
- cognitive performance

In other words, the heart can act as if it has a mind of its own and can profoundly influence the way you respond to the world. This program is based on this newly emerging view of the heart — the view that positive emotions lead to pain reduction, release of stress, better breathing and even better cognition.

It has been my experience that when a person involved with a crisis or traumatic loss is emotionally heard and deeply listened to, *all manner of things are possible.* I saw this over and over again in my work as a chaplain.

While working for hospice as a chaplain, I served a patient who had Parkinson's disease. He was unable to focus and couldn't often communicate beyond answering, "yes" and "no." His daughter was taking care of him — making arrangements for the nursing home, medical care, financial care and emotional care — really all aspects of life. The problem was twofold: First, the father was a mean, abusive alcoholic. The daughter was so angry that she could barely talk about her situation. It took great effort to be pleasant to her father. She was immensely bitter and consumed with distress over losing her freedom, support and happiness. I invited her to visit her father with me to speak her truth. My goal was to free her from the burden of her justified anger and sorrow. To my surprise, much more happened.

When we all met, I invited the father to accept his situation for what it was: the end-stage of life and the loss of his ability to talk easily. He was invited to grieve — and he moved into grief. He talked about his loss of mobility, speech and normalcy. I then invited the daughter to acknowledge her losses. She talked about her intense anger, her lost childhood and her current life of responsibility. This put them both on equal ground: They were both facing severe losses, were both angry and were both angry at one another.

Sharing this, they were invited to say a few words to each other. The daughter told her father how angry she was toward him, how abusive he had been and what a burden he had been in her life. I invited the father to say, "Would you forgive me?" And when the father said that, an ocean of grief came pouring out of the daughter. Some of her anger and bitterness subsided as she cried. She said she still loved him and that she was also angry at the life she led with him as a parent.

Each was then invited to say: "Thank you. I forgive you. Please forgive me. I love you."

As the daughter forgave, the father became more and more emotionally engaged and present. He began to speak using more words, longer phrases and fuller thoughts. He began to better comprehend her and tears appeared. As the father talked about the fears of his declining body, the magnitude of his terror became apparent. The daughter became more involved in the conversation. She too cried.

The father was able to see a blessing in his loss in that he had less to worry about now that life was simpler. For that he was grateful. And the daughter was grateful for the good material life her father had provided.

As prayers were offered, they moved into the bittersweet place where love and grief mingle. They sobbed together and seemed to recognize their mutual humanity and loss. They reached reconciliation and new emotional freedom to communicate. Each one's point of view broadened by listening to the other's grief. This was good for both of them, and it was good for the nursing staff that had to work with them.

This story is an example of engaging the heart's capabilities to move through loss, anger and grief to a place of balance and connection. Had we done this same exercise from the perspective of the mind, we would have ended up in an entirely different place. It has been my experience while working with hundreds of families facing death and loss that each of us has to make a choice: We can look at the loss from the point of view of the mind, or we can view the experience from the point of view of the heart. What I have witnessed is those who choose "the path of the open heart" are able to weave their way through sorrow and into deeper connection, community and love. It has also been my experience that those who choose "the way of the rational mind" end up in escalating cycles of criticism, blame, judgment and anger.

This program is based on choosing "the way of the open, wounded heart." Through it we go toward the despair, grief and sorrow. We wade around in its muddied waters to find new understandings and hope.

Please take five minutes to contemplate which choice you will make today: Do you want to try to resolve your sorrow from the perspective of the mind or the perspective of the heart? You have to make this choice; no one else can do it for you.

Let yourself relax into this question. Consider this from the point of view of your mind, and the point of view of your heart. Decide if you are willing to approach this program from your heart's perspective and let the rational, critical mind simply rest for a while.

It is my suggestion to revisit (if need be) your judgments, criticisms and recommendations later, while using this time now to give your heart a chance to grieve. If your choice at this point in time is to take the path of the rational mind, then I recommend that you put this aside for the moment and come back to it when you're feeling more receptive to your heart's perspective.

As you listen to your feelings, let yourself relax. Common feelings around loss include anxiety, fear, helplessness, anger, guilt or sorrow.

Anxiety or Fear

Sometimes, you may feel anxious or fearful. Often this comes from feeling helpless — feeling that you can't survive alone. Consider other adversities you have dealt with in your life. Remember how you handled those situations and consider applying some of those coping techniques now. Noticing the ways you have handled loss or adversity in the past can put these feelings into perspective. Include these feelings in your Candle-Lighting Prayer for this chapter.

Anger

Expressing anger, frustration or disappointment can be helpful to the grieving process. Many people experience anger in a situation involving loss. The anger is real and must go somewhere. If anger is not expressed, it may be turned inward and be experienced as depression, guilt or lowered self-esteem. Sometimes angry feelings come from intense pain. The pain could be physical or emotional. This is an excellent time to reflect on your anger and include it in your Candle-Lighting Prayer.

Guilt

There are a number of things that can cause feelings of guilt. You may regret choices you made regarding this loss situation. You may feel that you did not live up to your own standards, did not do enough or give enough. You may feel that you did not support your family emotionally. You may feel guilt over the actions of other people for their behavior. You may have made lifestyle choices that you now regret. You may have made choices that caused you to become ill. Whatever the reason for your feelings of guilt, you are invited to release these feelings in your Candle-Lighting Prayer.

Sorrow

It is appropriate to feel sorrow while you are going through (or recovering from) a loss. I encourage you to express whatever sorrow you have by writing it down, speaking it aloud and including it in your Candle-Lighting Prayer. The expression of sorrow can lead to clarity. Take some time now to consider what makes you sad ... and to what that sadness is connected. Consider how you would like to speak about this sorrow. Reflect on what is left unsaid that needs to be said now.

Scripture Readings

You are invited to read the following scripture aloud:

"I am ready to fall and my sorrow is continually before me."
— Psalm 38:17 and 13:2

Contemplation

Let yourself relax into your feelings to notice what you are feeling. Remember that "the way of the open heart" is toward the despair, grief and sorrow. See if you can find new understanding and hope.

Answer the following questions from your heart's point of view and write your answers in the space provided. Then as your heart expresses its regrets, notice the movement of your emotional energy and welcome that shift:

1. What feelings of loss live in you today?
2. What aspects or values from this situation (or person) do you accept as your own?
3. What aspects or values do you release?
4. What do you want to say that you could not say before?
5. What are you grieving from this loss?
6. What else can you release?
7. What can you forgive or understand?
8. Given what you are releasing and what you are keeping, what is the new perspective that you have now?
9. What have you learned, that you would not have learned without this loss?

Use this space to write down those feelings of loss that live in you today. Write down what you can release and what you need to say that you could not say before. At the end, describe your state of being after you have followed your heart's calling.

Please continue to the next page ...

Reflect on what you are learning. The main theme may be to "learn how to master discouragement" that comes from loss. The theme may be to "learn to let go of that which you love." Or, the theme may be "creating space for the next stage of your life." There are any number of themes for what can be learned from this loss.

Candle-lighting Prayer

The following prayer has been developed to support you as you name each feeling and offer it to God. The idea behind this prayer is to identify, name and release each feeling. As you present each feeling to God, keep the intention in your heart that "God will provide me with direction, wisdom and support for this process." Also, hold faith that in naming these feelings, there will be some movement toward new understanding and hope.

Recite these words aloud:

Gracious God and Sacred Holy Spirit

I give to You my judgments
and criticisms about this loss *(Light a candle.)*
To take, to hold, to transform.

I give to You my
Doubts, fears and anxieties *(Light a candle to represent these.)*
To take away.

I give to You my anger, shame, and frustration
Over this loss *(Light a candle.)*
To take, hold and transform.

It is my desire to follow the path
Of the open heart, to wade through
The swamp of sorrow, despair and pain
To come to a new place of understanding.
I light this candle now to represent
That intent and purpose
And ask that Your will prevail
To bring this purpose forward.

I grant You the authority to lead me
On this road despite my fears and doubts.
I pray for wisdom and understanding
And relief from this pain.
Please free my heart's love
For unrestricted movement away from these burdens
Please steady my feet on this path
Please guide my movement forward
That I may safely complete this journey
Into the land of gratitude, hope and understanding.

Chapter 6
How Others Impact Your Grief Process

"But there is no one who does not suffer, more or less secretly, from being in conflict with others and from being an agent of division rather than harmony among men, even though he is quite certain of being in the right."
— Paul Tournier

It would be such a blessing if every loss were accompanied by a designated time period of quiet, uninterrupted contemplation for those experiencing intense grief. In Western society, that is rarely (if ever) the case. Instead, it is common when coping with a loss to be dealing with other people who were present or involved in some way. And during a person's most sensitive or tender time, he or she may be forced to deal with emotionally charged matters of law, money or familial contention. Inevitably, some of the others involved will do things you find irritating, annoying or otherwise offensive. People tend to brood on these offenses, which only compounds the loss situation. In order to clear your heart, these irritations need to be released. The goal of this chapter is to support you in finding the will to embrace compassion, forgiveness and understanding.

The examples below may help you identify some of the ways "others" impacted your loss situation:

Loss of a loved one: If someone close to you died, it is possible that family members or friends said things that you experienced as painful. It is possible, even likely, that there were misunderstandings, grievances, arguments, disputes — even hostilities and confrontations. If you are a parent, spouse or sibling of someone who died in the hospital, you may have needed to interact with hospital administrators, doctors, nurses, discharge planners and perhaps social workers or spiritual support staff — in addition to other family members. And end-of-life situations may include funeral homes, attorneys, probate courts, financial trusts, investment bankers, debtors and relatives who are executors or hold power of attorney. You may hold resentments against some of those people involved or still be experiencing related anxiety of some kind.

Loss of employment: If you lost your job, you likely had to interface with human resources, coworkers, supervisors or unemployment/disability insurance personnel. Oftentimes, loss-of-employment situations also involve communication with affected family members.

Loss of property/other loss from natural disasters: Hurricanes, tornadoes, fires, floods and earthquakes require dealing with insurance companies, emergency workers, landlords, mortgage companies, neighbors, family members and perhaps reporting news media.

Loss of relationship/companionship/family bonds: When dealing with a loss of any kind, it is likely that some of the people involved have said things that hurt your feelings … or made suggestions that you did not take … or tried to push other people to do or think in a certain way about you and what happened. Maybe people became polarized and began to fight. Sometimes families will take sides and break apart during a loss; half will side with one person and half will side with the other.

It is not unusual to be ignored, rejected, ridiculed or misunderstood in situations of loss. You may feel upset by things that were said in a judgmental or critical manner. You may feel things were said or done in a personally denigrating or disrespectful way. The agenda of one faction may not correspond with your needs and feelings, and you may feel vulnerable as a result. In these situations, it can be hard to expel all those hurt feelings from inside you.

To successfully navigate a loss in which family members or factions became polarized is challenging. It is usually hard to stay on the path of the open heart in cases where family members or groups took sides. It is tempting to go into our rational minds and analyze what they said and did, then come up with judgments, criticisms and rationalizations about the whole thing. If you were in a situation where people became polarized, you are encouraged to approach the questions, scripture and prayers in this chapter with constant focus on *the feelings of your heart, rather than the thoughts of your mind.*

A word of warning: Once you start thinking too much about the things that people said and did, you'll find that you've detoured down "the path of the mind." At that point, just stop, back up and start over. If you find yourself going down that path, it might be more beneficial to just write down one item at a time and then do the Candle-Lighting Prayer for each of those items individually.

Laura is an example of someone who had to deal with others' accusations and recriminations. She was one of three adult children of an 89-year-old woman who had died.

Laura's experience was a common one for those dealing with an end-of-life situation: Many issues come up and decisions have to be made regarding the type and location of medical care, residential accommodations, daily caretaking, financial responsibility, selection of medical providers, management of real estate, execution of the will and burial arrangements. Laura and her sisters argued over these arrangements and who would be in charge of the decision-making process, even though the mother had designated Laura as the holder of Power of Attorney. Although Laura was the primary (and only) caretaker, her sisters accused her of neglecting her mother's care. They said this even though they lived out of town and never took the time to come and help.

Her sisters accused her of disregarding the doctor's orders because she moved her mother from a community hospital to a regional medical center with more sophisticated medical options. Her sisters accused her of mismanaging the estate because she hired a caretaker when her mother could no longer cook, clean and pay bills. Her sisters accused her of disregarding her mother's desires when she moved her mother to a retirement home where excellent hourly care was provided. And worst of all, her sisters said many untrue and hurtful things and tried to get the mother to turn against Laura.

Laura became despondent over the magnitude of the deception and the viciousness of the accusations. I met Laura after her mother had died and found that she was feeling deeply guilty. I invited her to examine these deceptions and accusations against the truth to determine if she was suffering from what Swiss physician and author Paul Tournier called *false guilt*. After many grief-counseling sessions together, Laura determined that it was not her guilt; she was carrying the guilt that her sisters would be carrying if they had understood the truth about the situation and understood all the careful work she was doing for her mother. Once she recognized this, she was able to release the *false guilt* and discovered new energy for her own life.

As you list the different people involved with your loss and what they said, it is possible you'll find there were collective social judgments or disapproval of your actions. It is possible that you carry guilt for not conforming to social norms and customs. This can happen when other people have expectations of how you should behave and you do not meet those expectations. When expectations go unmet, it can lead to judgment, criticism and blame.

If you are brooding over this kind of judgment, you may (like Laura) by carrying around *false guilt*. Feelings of *false guilt* can be examined to learn what they are based on and can be released if they come from self-accusations that have no foundation in fact. Specifically, this can occur when there were outright lies about you and your motives.

Even when you did not have the motives that were ascribed to you, if you still felt guilty, this is actually *false guilt.*

Tournier wrote in his book, *Guilt and Grace,* that in a crisis, people are all too ready to judge and condemn others with the moral certainty of God. They are all too ready to do this without inquiring beyond the surface to understand the complexities. They condemn you with overzealousness and rally others to join them. They go on a crusade to hold you responsible for some perceived error. They hope to bring you to your knees to confess responsibility for something you did not do — or did accidentally or unintentionally. They may claim to have the "absolute truth." They may conduct a vendetta to get others to treat you as an untouchable. It can become exhausting and even impossible to sort out the accusations, diversions and recriminations. This kind of conflict can escalate, leading to a permanent rift between you and the others.

Other times a *false guilt* hides a *true guilt*. This might occur when a family member blames you for the death of a loved one, even through you had no involvement in the death. Under this accusation you may be hiding a *true guilt* for not assuming more responsibility for the situation. This is when careful examination of your intentions and actions can be helpful.

Often, the various "guilts" mingle and overlap. But as we depend more on God and the Sacred, we may become freer of the disapproval of others and social pressures. This chapter offers you a chance to sort out where your feelings come from and then process and release them. Once you have clarified where they are coming from, you will be able to deal with them more easily.

Scripture Reading

You are invited to read the following scripture aloud:

"You should forgive and comfort him, otherwise one might be overwhelmed by excessive sorrow."

— 2 Cor 2:7

Contemplation

One way to navigate through the anguish and misery arising from other people's troublesome behavior is to reconnect with your core purpose and the bigger view of events and circumstances. It can be a struggle to release this type of anguish and suffering because it was so personal. But as you gain clarity on the magnitude and number of people, agencies and organizations involved — and the variety of the different agendas — you will begin to realize the range of perspectives from which the other parties were operating.

The goal is to make peace with the variants between their point of view and your point of view. The more that you can sit and contemplate, "What was this like for them?" the easier it's going to be for you to step back and take the galactic, big-picture perspective on the loss. This more distant perspective comes as you consider the agendas and needs and goals of all the other parties involved. And then, as you consider your own needs and goals in light of those of all these other parties, your perspective will broaden and your heart will have a better chance of releasing its hurt.

The focus of this chapter is to move to the galactic perspective. The first step in this direction is to list the different groups that were involved, review their point of view and consider how theirs differs from your point of view. Take time to contemplate each point of view side-by-side to your own. Let yourself consider them together in one mind and at the same time. Consider what you can release and what you need to hold onto. Write your answers in the space provided.

The goal is to find your will for compassion, forgiveness and understanding from the galactic perspective. To reach that goal, the following questions may be helpful:

1. Who supported you? Who did not support you?
2. What was said that hurt you?
3. What was done that offended you?
4. What can you forgive and release?
5. What do you need to hold on to?
6. What is your heart's point of view at this time?
7. What is your spirit's point of view at this time?
8. What new understanding has this brought out in your heart and spirit?

List the different groups involved. Review their point of view and consider how theirs differs from yours. Take time to contemplate each point of view side-by-side to your own. Consider what you can release and what you need to hold onto at this time:

_____
_____
_____
_____
_____
_____
_____
_____
_____
_____
_____
_____
_____
_____
_____
_____
_____
_____
_____

Please continue to the next page …

Candle-Lighting Prayer

Now that you have identified people involved in this loss and identified what they said and did that pained or irritated you, it is time for your Candle-Lighting Prayer. Light a candle for each person and experience you wish to release from your heart. Give yourself enough time to allow your heart to be clear and your grief to move into new energy.

Recite these words aloud:

Sovereign God
I open myself to Your will and love
To be transformed this day from sorrow to wisdom.

Source of creation
I honor You as the source of all
I honor Your truth and goodness

Source of life
Source of peace
I acknowledge Your peace

Source of mercy
Source of strength, I acknowledge Your mercy;
I lean on You for courage.

Creative God of all being
Bring my spirit into Your presence
Align my hopes with Yours

Giver of love
Prepare me to receive and know Your good and perfect gifts
To open my hearts to Your love

Searcher of hearts
Illuminate my sorrows
Remind me of Your glory

Sacred Holy Spirit
Come enfold my will to
Reconcile with others
Who may have been misinformed,
And mistaken about my intentions, actions, words.

Come lead me into recognizing
The point of view of others
The expectations of others
That feel unreasonable. *(Light a candle.)*

By lighting these candles
I release my grievances, conflicts
Disputes, confrontations and
Misunderstandings. *(Light a candle.)*

Guide my heart to relinquish
The pain and disappointment
Over what was said and done
By others *(Light a candle for each person.)*

I lift up unfounded accusations to be released into Your care.
I lift up deception about my motives to be released into Your care.
I lift up condemnation for errors that I did not commit.
I lift up what was done accidentally and unintentionally
To be released into Your care. *(Light candles.)*

I lift up dishonesty deceit and fabrication,
Fraud, pretexts, and ruses
Resentment and anger
Held by myself and others to be released into Your care.
I release all this to You and ask for consolation, comfort
and nurturing from Your all-knowing spirit
and gracious love. *(Light a candle.)*

Source of truth
I seek to know truth in the midst of loss
I seek the fine wisdom encased in our sorrows
Source of all true joy
May I receive Your blessing in this work today
and return to joy again.

I dedicate this time to this end in your name and will.

Chapter 7
The Soul's Perspective on Your Suffering

"You can hold yourself back from the suffering of the world: this is something you are free to do... but perhaps precisely this holding back is the only suffering you might be able to avoid."

— Franz Kafka

In this chapter, you are invited to look at your loss from "the soul's point of view." There are various ideas about what the soul's point of view is. One view is that the soul is the vital, passionate part of you that feels love, hate, grief and joy. According to this view, you could look at your loss in terms of how it impacted your ability to experience these passionate feelings.

An alternative view is that the soul is the part of the Self that develops moral values and has the ability to distinguish between good and evil. This view asks you to look at your loss in terms of how it helped you develop moral values and the ability to distinguish between good and evil.

A third view of the soul is that it is the part of you that enjoys and acknowledges the existence and presence of God. According to this view, you undergo loss for the purpose of becoming purified, in order to become aware of the Divine life force itself. This is the part of the soul that can achieve a full union with God. This view asks you to look at loss in terms of how you became purified and how your awareness of the Divine life force increased.

A fourth view is that the soul watches from outside the physical and material plane. This view is concerned with expansion to a broader perspective and sees your entire life in terms of how a loss helped you to understand and speak your own truth, build compassion for others or grow in wisdom.

Whichever definition you choose to use, remember that the soul looks at a bad situation and sees it as worthwhile — as worth a pot of gold.

I once met a homeless man at a hospital who was miserable. I asked him what was making him so unhappy, and he told me that he was lonely. I knew that he had doctors and nurses coming in every few minutes who were very interested in him, so I asked him if he was feeling some friendship with them. He disagreed. They *were* the problem, he said.

They came in all day long extracting blood and taking samples and talking about his body and his temperature and his illness. But he felt that they did not really care about him. I asked him what caring would look like and learned that what he wanted was to have a soulful conversation with someone. He wanted to talk about the meaning of life, not about his body temperature, blood work or prognosis. As I talked with him more, I learned that his highest value was to speak the truth and to know and understand people at the deepest level. He wanted to have a soulful conversation with the nurses and doctors, but they were not available for that. He longed for a soul friend, such as his homeless friends whose singular focus was to speak of the deepest truths about themselves.

This was a man who lived in the way of the soul.

When I discovered how bright he was, I asked him why he didn't have a regular life with a job and a place to live. He said that didn't interest him because it did not feed his soul. He was finding his life of homelessness offered access to soulfulness, and that he did not want to give this up. His soul's view of homelessness was that it offered him a valuable lifestyle because it fostered speaking the truth, hearing the truth and forged deep understanding with others.

This story demonstrates how a person's soul might have an unusual point of view that is healing and hopeful. This man needed his soul's point of view in order to deal with the unfamiliar people and procedures at the hospital. Just as he needed to find his soul's point of view, so do you. Based on the previously mentioned ways that the soul might look at loss, you are invited to consider your own loss situation.

From the soul's perspective, this loss may be an invitation to shift your perspective to your underlying passions and ask what value was gained by this increase in passion.

From the soul's perspective, this loss may be an invitation to shift your perspective to new moral values and ask how this loss informs your understanding of good and evil.

From the soul's perspective, this may be an opportunity to discover how this loss helped you purify yourself for the sake of engaging with the Divine life force.

From the soul's perspective, this may be an invitation to ask how this loss helped you to understand and speak your own truth, build compassion for others or grow in wisdom.

You are invited to focus on your "soul's potential" in the loss situation you have experienced. In every crisis there is the potential for the soul to expand. Your work is to contemplate your soul's potential in this loss — to find that and claim it. Contemplate your soul's point of view as you faced this loss, this pathology or this enemy.

Look to see if there was a structural shift in your passions, moral values, wisdom or connection with God.

To explore this, try listening to music and let your imagination open to the flow of memories, hopes, desires and regrets. Look at this situation within the context of your entire life. See your life as being at the service of your imagination, so that what you carry in your imagination informs your soul of the meaning of things. Try turning the facts upside-down. You could do this by saying to yourself: "What was the soul's wisdom in this situation?" … "What was the golden lesson to be learned?" … "What would not have happened to me if this situation had not occurred?" … "What essential core idea, value, shift or change took place as a result of this event?"

Look at the loss upside-down. Look at your sorrow and wounds from the point of view of how it challenged your essential traits or practices. Ask yourself what this situation wanted from you and what it called forth in you. Ask yourself what it did to you, where it took you, and what it took from you.

When my own mother was sick with Alzheimer's and things became chaotic, my rational mind told me to walk away; that the situation was too unreasonable and that all my efforts were fruitless. Every time I went there to see her, she had forgotten that I came to see her the day before. She'd be angry and would say, "You don't ever help me."

As you might imagine, this was an intolerable situation for me. Every time I went to see her, I felt guilty all over again. And yet, the guilt was irrational because I had actually been there the day before! *In fact, I had been there 30-hours-a-week for a whole year.* So, from the point of view of my rational mind, this situation was unmanageable, and the logical conclusion was to extract myself from the situation. But on the other hand, after five years of hanging in there with her and offering her support and service, my soul began to feel a sense of satisfaction at the work I was doing and the service I was providing. It didn't matter if it was appreciated or not. It was just satisfying to my soul. And actually, I realized 10 years later that I had grown and that my soul had changed direction and become much more interested in service because of how satisfying that experience was — even if on a certain level it was irrational.

Scripture Reading

You are invited to read the following scripture aloud:

> "My sorrow is beyond healing and my heart is faint within me."
>
> — Jer 8:18

Contemplation

Take some time to clarify the situation. The following questions are designed to help you identify you soul's perspective on this loss. Write down in the space provided the ways that your soul might look at this loss situation. Select a focus for today. Review the feelings that are connected to this loss:

1. What understanding does your soul have with regard to this loss?
2. In what ways might your soul grow in understanding this loss?
3. Examples of the soul's perspectives might include:
   - Building depth and compassion
   - Moral learning
   - Character building
   - Shifted community alignment
   - Shifted financial orientation
   - Shifted personality
   - Reconnection with God
   - Changed boundaries
   - New vistas
   - Courage
   - Wisdom
4. Imagine that the bindings on your soul are released, your soul is rising and you can see farther from a galactic point of view. What is your soul's new point of view on this loss?

Use this space to clarify the situation:

Please continue to the next page ...

Candle-Lighting Prayer for the Soul's Journey

This prayer encourages you to release expectations from your heart, see the "bigger picture" and go deeper.

Recite these words aloud:

Gracious God, Sacred Spirit

Praise Your all-knowing illumination
Praise Your graceful ways
Praise Your glory and mercy.

Open me to deeper knowing
Bring forth broader vision
Lead my imagination to new possibilities
Guide my journey through this dark night.

What emptiness is this?
What is absolved, forgiven, excused?
What arid, parched, bone-dry place is this?
Edify the value of this affliction and darkness

Take this suffering and pain
Tutor me past expectations, desires
Instruct me in this upside-down disarray
Guide me on a journey from darkness into light

Show me what gains my soul
Traveling down this painful road
What passion, purity, what truth, what wisdom
Can bring forth from grief to gratitude.

Chapter 8
What You Need to Know about Loss of Self

"My joy is gone, grief is upon me, my heart is sick."
— Jeremiah 8.18

There are a number of different ways you can *lose yourself* when you go through a traumatic loss, life-changing circumstance or loss of a loved one. The first way is to lose your values, hopes, energy or focus. The second way is through neglect and poor self-care. The third way is to lose yourself by way of being unable or unwilling to act according to your own standards. The fourth way is to give away your skills or values to another person.

Let's examine these one at a time:

Loss of Parts of Self

The first type of *loss of Self* is common during the long-term care of someone who is terminally ill. It is not unusual to discover that when the loved one dies, you have lost part of yourself. This can happen because you gave a lot of yourself to the relationship and to the other person during the course of the relationship. You may have made certain sacrifices to be with that person. Those sacrifices include your time and energy, and you may have even given up some of your interests and values for the sake of the loved one. The situation may have required you to give up parts of yourself in order to be present to the overriding needs of the person. When you discover what parts of yourself are missing or submerged, it can be energizing to reclaim them.

You may have given up having your needs met or your priorities fulfilled or your values honored in any one of the following areas:

- Friends and family
- Health
- Money
- Career
- Physical environment
- Fun and recreation
- Personal growth
- Romance

Other aspects that became submerged or temporarily lost during this experience might include:

- Your "Playful Self"
- Your "Vulnerable Self"
- Your "Creative Self"
- Your "Adult Self"
- Your Self-esteem and Self-worth
- Your "Carefree Self"
- Your "Peaceful Self"
- Your "Joyful Self"

In the space provided, write down some parts of yourself that have been neglected, submerged or repressed as a result of this loss.

Neglect of Self

During an extended loss that goes on for months or years (such as caring for an elderly parent, spouse or sibling, or recovering from a loss of work, health, home or support system), it is helpful to notice how well you took care of yourself. Taking care of someone or something over a long period of time can be not only exhausting, it can be distracting. There is so much to do. You might be dealing with medical care, physical care, financial care, friends and family, personal growth and recreational activities, just to name a few. You may have forgotten to take care of your own health and nutrition or neglected your own friendships and personal relationships. You may have forgotten to get enough emotional support or tend to responsibilities other than those relating to your loss situation. You may have simply forgotten to have fun and get enough rest. If there were ways in which you neglected to take care of yourself, write them down in the space provided.

Loss of Standards

Sometimes people under stress are unable to live up to their own standards, ideals or abilities. In a sudden and traumatic situation this can happen. And when this happens, it is possible to carry a vague sense of guilt. This guilt comes from letting yourself down —knowing you could have offered more (or wanted to offer more) than you did in the situation. This feeling can be dealt with by releasing yourself from self-criticism, blame and judgment.

Close your eyes for a moment and imagine you are an attorney defending a client ... and that client is *you*. List all the extenuating circumstances that made it impossible for you to live up to all these expectations.

For example: Grief and shock paralyzed you. The magnitude of the situation was overwhelming, and you became so anxious you were unable to use all your skills. Perhaps other people's strong words, actions or interventions stopped you from exercising good judgment. Maybe your desire to be accepted by other people kept you from confrontation and disagreement. Or, inability to confront bad behavior created a sense of guilt of being inadequate. Write down the standards and abilities that you did not live up to in the space provided.

Things You Took On & Things You Gave Away

Alternatively, just as you gave up some needs or values in a relationship, you have also taken some of the other person's interests, priorities or values into yourself. By taking on their interests, pastimes, activities as if they were you own, you have taken parts of them into you. Now that the person has passed away or moved on, it is time to look at what you took on. It is time to decide what you want to keep, and what you want to return to your loved one. Write these things down in the space provided.

While working as a chaplain, I visited a man in the hospital whose leg had just been amputated. His wife was comforting him at his bedside, but she was also telling him "not to cry," and that "it would be okay." As I was talking to him, she kept interrupting him and telling him not to cry. I began to realize that she was interfering in his grieving process about the loss of his leg, and I actually asked her to leave the room.

After she left, I asked the man what kind of pain he was experiencing. It turned out that he was feeling emotional pain, not physical pain. He was in deep despair about the loss of his leg and the change of lifestyle this loss would entail. So, I invited him to grieve the loss by talking about it, weeping and telling me all the things that he was going to miss and all his regrets and sorrows.

The man regretted all the activities, people and events that would no longer be in his life. He believed that his friends would forsake him. He believed that his lifelong hobbies would be lost and that nothing new would replace them. He feared that he would be homebound for the rest of his life and go back to drinking again. He was bereft over the lost parts of his life, the lost friends and loss of lifelong activities as a result of the amputation of his leg.

We spent about an hour together grieving, and at the end of that time, he fell asleep. I later learned that prior to our meeting, he hadn't slept for 36 hours. This was in part because his wife was striving very hard to repress his grief process.

The next day, she told me how much better he felt, how well he had slept and how glad they were that he was able to take the time to grieve the loss of his leg.

This story exemplifies how before grieving, a situation can look and feel hopeless, but afterward, the circumstances seem manageable and hope can return.

Scripture Reading

You are invited to read the following scripture aloud:

"I was mute and silent; I kept silent and refrained even from good
And my sorrow grew worse."

— Psalm 39:2

Contemplation

Reflect on the aspects of yourself that became submerged or temporarily lost during this experience. Consider ways you may have neglected to take care of yourself or were unable to live up to your standards. Were there any needs or values that you gave up or lost?

1. What guilt do you have about yourself in relation to yourself during this loss situation?
2. What aspects of yourself have you neglected during this loss?
3. What aspects of yourself have you fulfilled during this loss?
4. What values did you give away?
5. What values that you gave away do you want to reclaim?
6. What values did you acquire?
7. What values that you received would you like to release now?
8. What strength or wisdom did you gain during this time?
9. What new understanding does this bring to you now?

Write down parts of yourself that were neglected. Write down ways that you neglected yourself. Write down any ways that you failed to live up to your own standards:

_____
_____
_____
_____
_____
_____
_____
_____
_____
_____
_____
_____
_____
_____
_____
_____
_____
_____
_____
_____

Please continue to the next page ...

Candle-Lighting Prayer

Select some key aspects of the things that you want to release during this prayer. In this prayer, you will state your needs, thank yourself for having given up those needs (for the blessing of the relationship) and welcome those needs back into your life again. Things you took on may also be released in the following prayer.

Recite these words aloud:

Wise and Gracious God,
Lover of goodness,
Giver of blessings,
Beloved force of transformation,
Holder of griefs and losses
May Your blessed presence oversee this prayer.

God of all history,
God of all time,
God of all futures,
I am in emotional turmoil with this loss.
Lead the way forward in my life.

Giver of blessings, direct me in reclaiming losses:
Lost Self, lost standards, lost values and lost abilities.
Reverse my self-negligence, desertion and disregard
Repair my abandonment, inattention and lack of care,
Transform these into comprehension, discernment and perception.

Guide me through the *Loss of Self* in these areas:
(State what they are, light a candle for each one and say: "I present my loss of Self in its many forms for guidance and transformation.")

Loving God, guide my heart to accept these losses
Transformed into emotional growth and profound wisdom
Becoming a new foundation
A source of joy and abundance;
I invite You gracious God, to advance this cause.

Creator of all new things, I honor *Self Renewal*
I reclaim my *lost Self, lost standards, lost values.*
I call forth self-acceptance, tolerance, support
I welcome Your lavish understanding

I invite an abundant life with a full Self present
Welcome abundant Grace
My heart is open to You this day.
I reclaim my *lost Self* and
Welcome Your vigor and energy.

God, thank you for blessing this prayer
May I receive Your blessing well
May I take Your blessing to reflect, pray and weep
May I notice and be comforted by Your grace.

Chapter 9
How Inner Conflicts Perpetuate Grief

"The meeting with oneself is the meeting with one's own shadow. To mix a metaphor, the shadow is a tight pass, a narrow door, whose painful constriction is spared to no one who climbs down into the deep wellspring. But one must learn to know oneself in order to know who one is."

— Carl Jung

There is an idea that we are made up of many selves. Think of a loss in which part of you rejoiced and part was utterly disappointed. These two feelings represent valid parts of you, each with different needs. The goal of this chapter is to identify these inner conflicts — to uncover them and give them room to be expressed. This is an essential step in grieving because each part of you has a valid point of view, and getting through your grief will require you to deal with this reality.

During a major loss, conflicts occur not only with other people but also from within. For example, one part of you might be angry, while another part might be ashamed. One part might feel guilty, while another part might feel anxious. One part of you might be fearful, while another part is relieved. This chapter is focused on making peace between the conflicting parts of yourself.

Exhaustion and fatigue are signs that an inner conflict is at work. For example, a man lost his job and part of him was embarrassed and ashamed. But another part of him rejoiced to be free again. (He was too tired to go out and get another job because of this inner, unresolved conflict.)

Another example might be a father who carries anger over his son's death because the son was drinking or doing drugs. In addition to anger, the father might feel guilty because he didn't stop his son in time or didn't teach him differently. And that father might feel shame about what other people think — or shame about not being a good enough (or an absent) parent. He might have anxiety that his other children will follow in the same footsteps, be fearful that the authorities will accuse him of neglect or feel relieved when the funeral is over (because he no longer has to supervise a wayward child).

The sooner the father works with these conflicting emotions, the sooner he will be able to release his grief.

Another example of conflicts within came up while I was working with a man who had divorced his wife. He had a great deal of conflict about the divorce. "The Protector" in him was angry because she had gotten involved with another man. "The Adult" felt guilty for having neglected his marriage. His "Inner Child" was fearful to be alone again. And "The Adventurer" in him was relieved that he could start over and find someone who was a better match.

As he worked with all these different energies and began to own them fully, he was able to look at them and grieve for each part of himself that was distressed over this massive change in his life. By lighting a candle for each part and taking the time to contemplate each feeling, he was able to make significant inroads in releasing the intense knot that was preventing him from moving forward in his life. By very methodically working on each one of these feelings and parts, he gradually got through his grief and was able to release these intense feelings.

Once the intensely complicated, interwoven feelings were sorted out, he was able to take in a broader view and new perspective on his situation. He arrived at the conclusion that there were a number of significant parts of him that had not been met or acknowledged in his marriage, and now he was ready and able to search for a life partner who could satisfy some of his deeper needs. And in this way, the loss became a blessing. He realized that although he had lost something he valued, he was hopeful because he had room for something new that could be potentially even more valuable.

Scripture Reading

You are invited to read the following scripture aloud:

> "I have great sorrow and unceasing grief in my heart."
>
> — Romans 9:2

Contemplation

Take some time to consider the conflicts within that are expressing different needs and feelings. Use this time to name the conflicts within and give them space to be fully expressed and validated:

1. List some parts of yourself that are in conflict over this loss.
2. Explore the part of you that is the "rational mind" and the part of you that is the "aching heart."
3. Are these two parts in conflict over your loss? If so, how?
4. Contemplate and validate each part's needs and feelings.
5. What part is the loudest? What part is silent or barely audible?
6. Imagine rebalancing your energy to distribute it more equally among the parts.
7. What is the optimal balance between parts, and how is this different?
8. Imagine holding a new center of balance between these parts of yourself.
9. What new understanding do you have now about your optimal center of balance?

On this page, write down the conflicts you notice. What part of you is in conflict with another part of yourself?

Please continue to the next page ...

Candle-Lighting Prayer for the Reconciliation of Conflicts

This chapter is focused on the discovery and acceptance of the conflicting parts of yourself. During this releasing prayer, you are invited to come to peace with these conflicting needs and feelings.

Consider for a moment the conflicting parts of yourself. Contemplate in your heart the depth of the feelings around this emotion. During this prayer, light a candle for each conflicting part of yourself, and have the goal of releasing it when you light the candle. As you contemplate your feelings, you are invited to weep. And weep as long as you need to, then forgive yourself.

At the end of this prayer, take some time to look at those multiple conflicting parts of yourself from a different point of view.

- The part of you that's angry might have been "The Protector."
- The part that's ashamed might have been "The Child" in you.
- The part that's guilty might be "The Parent."
- The part that's angry might be "The Adult."
- The part that's relieved might be "The Career Professional."

Light a set of candles representing all these parts of yourself and say a prayer for each part of yourself.

As you conclude the Candle-Lighting Prayer, you will have honored and acknowledged conflicting parts of yourself.

You will have given them over to God for caretaking.

Look at this situation from the galactic point of view.

You are invited to mull over what you've learned from this experience.

See if you have found a broader and deeper perspective on your life.

Recite these words aloud:

Lord, please hear this prayer.
Be a shepherd to me in my
Journey of reconciliation.

Introduce me to the ways
Of the Holy Spirit who
Miraculously removes, releases, transforms
Suffering into wisdom.

Shepherd and guide each part of myself
To understand the ways of forgiveness.
Guide my mind, heart, and spirit
To unified understanding
Of the truth of this path and
The value of this journey.

I give over to You these conflicts
Simmering within myself:
(List the conflicts you have while lighting a candle for each one.)

I forgive each part of myself
I have suffered enough.
I am tired and worn out with strife
I release all resentment toward myself
Into the care of Your Holy Spirit.

Guide me safely through
Nights of anger and swamps of sorrow
Past the trees of regret
Into meadows of love
Upon the rock of the soul,
To behold the wide skies of faith,
With God's Glory.

Chapter 10
Why a New Perspective Leads to Transformation

"Every now and then, life takes us in a big leap forward, sometimes, it seems, by the scruff of our necks."

— Molly Young Brown

Transformation comes out of crisis and vulnerability. This chapter encourages you to see the crisis in your life as a source of revelation. You are invited to view your loss as a doorway into a perspective that is broader, deeper and more compassionate. The questions and prayers in this chapter are to help you reflect on how this crisis has changed your feelings, thoughts or beliefs.

Take a few moments to review your notes from each preceding chapter. Track the changes you went through as you examined each element of your loss. As you do this, allow some emotional room to see that conflict, despair and anguish are an integral part of the transformation through which you are now going. Make a connection between the anguish and your change in perspective. Notice how they need each other, feed each other and are a part of each other. You are invited to reflect on the idea that your broader, deeper perspective comes out of the anguish.

During a crisis, the deficiencies in the situation, yourself or in others become apparent and lead you to alternative ways of thinking. At a time like this, conflicts in your values, beliefs and practices are stressful and maybe even threatening. But these conflicts can also move you toward revitalizing new possibilities. These possibilities come with new understandings of the way things are — or the way you want them to be (and the way to live). The fastest way through grief is to clarify these value conflicts and acknowledge new possibilities.

As the gap between the ideal and the real becomes wider, the crisis feels more intense. Whatever the crisis, your spirit seeks relief from pain and a new way of being in the world. Your task is to make an emotional shift or to find a new way of being or new values.

The grieving process leads to a variety of changes such as the rejection of old beliefs and search for new beliefs and values. You discover that you have been on a quest that has driven you to go beyond where you are to find a new worldview and system of meaning. This involves letting go of certain things and making space for a new perspective.

The deeper you go into the meaning of your grief, the more responsibility you will assume for your emotions and desires. The process of examining all aspects of your emotional life — including grief, anger, panic, shame, guilt and acceptance — challenges you to grow emotionally. The result can lead to a change in personal affiliations, emotional or lifestyle priorities, family priorities and your relationship to God.

An example of this is a woman I met who was suicidal. It was about 10 o'clock at night when I was called to the bedside of a woman who said she did not want to go on with her life. It turned out that she'd been bedridden for the past six years and was living in a group home. And it was clear that she was going to have to go back to that group home and continue living her life in bed.

The immediate problem was she wasn't getting well during her stay at the hospital, and that seemed to be related to her despair over her life prospects. I began talking with her and learning more about her and her situation. I discovered that despite her circumstances, she seemed to be serving as a chaplain to the other patients in the convalescent hospital. It was true that she might be bedridden, but she was still doing a important work; she was listening deeply to these people and showing up for them. I explained that was a tremendous service because she was listening to their hearts and souls and feeding their life force by doing this deep listening.

We continued to talk, and eventually I came to ask her what she thought her calling in life was. She thought about it, and then she said her calling was to give support, encouragement and affirmation to her roommates at the group home (who also all had chronic medical conditions requiring 24/7 convalescent care). I asked her what she had given to people and what she had received from people over the years. She replied that she had given a lot of support and hope, and she had received a lot of gratitude and affirmation, and that it was all very satisfying to her. She said it felt like this work was her life mission. As she talked about these things, her point of view shifted. She began to feel more satisfaction over the life she had lived and began to honor the support and service that she had given.

Before she got to this place, however, she did quite a bit of grieving and weeping over the loss of life potential and the loss of hope of ever having a normal life. And I think it was the connection between the grieving and the weeping and the searching for her life's mission that helped her release her sorrow and rededicate herself to this life of service as a patient in a convalescent care facility.

The point of this story is that when you link your grieving to your life purpose (or life service), you can reframe the loss in a way that helps you let go of it. And so, that's what you're invited you to do now — to remember who you are, what your calling is and what your service in this life is.

There are many ways that your perspective might shift after going through a great loss. For example, a woman who had been married 34 years lost her husband to cancer. Her life had revolved around her home, family and husband's career. After his death, she took up photography and traveled the world as a photo journalist. She became more aware of different cultures and lifestyles. Her interests shifted from homemaking to art, culture and politics.

It is not unusual for a significant loss to lead to a decision to give up one career for another. I once met a wealthy businessman who was hospitalized for a long time. During his hospitalization, he decided to leave the business world for international service work with non-profits in undeveloped countries. This loss created an opening for new life vistas.

Another example is a son who was one of five siblings who had durable Power of Attorney for the healthcare of his father. The father was hospitalized with end-stage renal disease, and the doctors wanted this son to make a decision about whether to perform additional medical treatments that would prolong the father's life ... but only by a few weeks and with a decrease in quality of life. The siblings were divided for and against this decision. The son's decision over whether to "resuscitate" his father every time he was declining, took courage. As a result of this experience, his character expanded with newfound understanding of courage.

Another fellow lost his job because he disliked his coworkers. He was a sports enthusiast and his coworkers were computer geeks interested in software engineering. This fellow saw the world in "black and white." He believed that there was something wrong with the guys who were not interested in sports. He became hostile to his coworkers and was uncooperative. After loosing his job, he realized that he needed to expand his tolerance quotient for other people's opinions and preferences. This is a situation where loss resulted in building more tolerance in his character.

Another situation was the group of siblings who were fighting over how to best care for elderly parents with senile dementia and cancer. One sibling was a creative artist who was not very experienced with "practical" matters. Another sibling was a businessman who was used to "controlling the outcome." Another sibling was intimately involved in the daily caretaking but had sacrificed her own life boundaries. In order to work together (or even to make a contribution to caring for their parents), each one had to shift their perspective: The artist had to come to grips with practical realities and make room for practical decisions — even when they were contrary to aesthetic values. The businessman had to learn to listen to others' opinions and negotiate through differences. The caretaking sibling had the opportunity to expand her perspective from pure service to look at the situation from other perspectives.

In any situation of loss, there usually is an opportunity to shift or expand one's perspective. This could be from academic to practical, from objective to subjective, from fun to "meaningful," from mainstream to creative, from business to service, from planning to spontaneous. In a loss situation, there is usually an opportunity to build character. You might learn the courage to stand up for what you believe, to let go of absolutist thinking, to tolerate other people's opinions, to honor other people's viewpoints, to be collaborative or to state your feelings and needs. Often a loss will help you to clarify your core values.

This chapter is dedicated to finding your will to wholeness and finding the faith to trust God — all with an open expression of suffering, rather than deny your suffering. The result is the discovery of new perspectives on grief. See what new perspectives you can find as you consider your losses.

Scripture Reading

You are invited to read the following scripture aloud:

> "God heals the broken hearted and binds up their sorrows."
>
> — Psalm 143:3

Contemplation

Reflect on what this loss has opened up for you. Think about your original perspectives. Consider new perspectives that are coming forward. If none come forward, try another point of view. Take some time now to reflect on the ways this loss has changed or contributed to your character, values and convictions. Consider how your orientation has changed. Consider how this loss has impacted your understanding of the way you want to live.

1. How has your perspective on this loss been altered by family or friends?
2. How has this loss affected your perspective on work?
3. How has your value for leisure time and recreation been impacted by this loss?
4. How has your financial perspective shifted as a result of this loss?
5. How has your value for personal growth been impacted by this loss?
6. How has your perspective on your living situation shifted as a result of this loss?
7. What new perspectives have you see as a result of this loss?

After a few moments, contemplate one final question from the point of view of your heart, soul and spirit:

"What would be absent from my life now had this loss not occurred?"

As you examine your loss and answer these questions, write down how your perspective has been challenged or changed in these arenas: family and friends, work, recreation and fun, finances, personal growth, living situation and connection to God. Notice how your point of view changes as you search for your answers:

_____
_____
_____
_____
_____
_____
_____
_____
_____
_____
_____
_____
_____
_____
_____
_____
_____
_____
_____
_____
_____

Please continue to the next page ...

Candle-Lighting Prayers for Mourning Losses & Welcoming New Perspectives

Take a few minutes to reflect on the sorrow you are experiencing. Light a candle for each of these griefs. When you light the candle, say this prayer and ask God to bring forth a new perspective. Take time to reflect on each grief to see if you can discover new understanding. See if there is an emotional or mental shift in how you are holding this grief. At the end of the prayer, light a candle for whatever shift has occurred in your thinking. Notice the impact of this prayer over the next several days and weeks. Look for a change in perspective to come forward in subtle ways. Open your heart to receive this gift.

Recite these words aloud:

Come my God, and mourn with me
Come my God, and inspect my grief
Come my God, and heal my sorrow

Awaken my heart with the fire of Your love
Inspire my spirit with the strength of Your mind
Provoke my soul with the force of Your vision

I confess I have lost sight of wisdom
The wisdom of my original state
The wisdom of Your great love
The wisdom of understanding.

I confess I have lost some compassion
The compassion for my beliefs
The compassion for my values
The compassion for my practices.

I confess I have great anguish over this loss
With a churning and mulling mind
Over what I desired and what transpired
Over what was said and done and undone.

Gracious Loving God, I request that You
Guide me toward gratitude and creativity
To make sense of the space between the ideal and the real
Carry me through this change of perspective

Beloved Loving God, I invite You to
Shift my bearing, posture and direction,
To bring forth a new emotional wisdom
To hold deeper meaning and value.

God of Joy and Peace
Release the old to bring forth
New understanding, perspectives and vistas
With broad and deep illumination.

Take a few minutes to remember what you are grateful for that your loved one gave you or that was given to you by your life circumstances. Light a candle to acknowledge these things for which you are grateful.

If at this time you have seen that gratitude is the way to joy — if you have found a connection with spirit — reflect on the possibilities.

Consider this reflection as a path to a new perspective.

At times you may have felt that your losses have made a barren landscape of your life. You may have felt that this loss has taken away your ability to see the mountains you have climbed.

You are invited to take a look around you and see that you can soar above the mountains … and see how small they look from your new perspective.

Chapter 11
The Art of Grieving

"The one reality to which we ultimately belong and which therefore most intimately belongs to us can be called God."

— David Steindl-Rast

At the very least, the expression and release of grief can lead to a sense of balance and authenticity. At best, it can lead to an unveiling of your life purpose, revision of your core values and a shift in your understanding of life's meaning. My hope is that you will experience elements of each of these aspects as you complete Chapter 11.

The goal of this chapter is to help you discover a sense of connection (with yourself, with others and with God) that is relevant, authentic, renewing, moving and peaceful. It has been my experience that as people find greater connection with themselves, they are better able to access passion in their life. This frees up new energy and cuts through the numbness that people often experience when they first lose someone or something of value.

As people find greater connection with others, they begin to move back into the flow of life, to socialize with friends and get involved in stimulating activities. And as people find greater connection with God, they discover new pathways to intuition, mystery and the Sacred. This in turn creates space for joy, hope and possibility in life.

It has been my experience that at some point, people begin to understand the *Art of Grieving*. The *Art of Grieving* is the recognition that it takes an irritation to make a pearl out of an oyster.

You may have gone through a long, barren time of finding no solace, support or comfort. You may have been overpowered by the massiveness of circumstances with a weight and force that dampened your spirit. You may have felt that this caused you such pain that you lost your desire to move forward. I would like to suggest that in the midst of this emptiness, this darkness, this pain and suffering, you are in a special place. This is the place where the Divine and human meet and open into the realm of wonder, wisdom and love.

This period of darkness that you have gone through has created an opportunity to open your heart, spirit and soul to Divine Love. The road for this journey is prayer and contemplation. Weeping combined with prayer and contemplation of the sacred aspects of your loss illuminates the path of understanding. By traveling down this road, it is possible to move into deeper levels of self-care and self-respect, broadened acceptance of others and a magnified receptivity to sacred ways of knowing. By traveling down this road, you invite Divine light into your spirit, and this creates an opportunity for unleashing and releasing. This process includes weeping, praying and listening for understanding. This process invites the possibility of transformation of loss into wisdom. By undertaking this process, you are making the courageous decision to journey through the dark into understanding and love.

You have courageously entered into the darkness of yourself, of others, of the situation; this has no doubt been painful. But this is the path that purges you of inner and outer conflicts, inner and outer resentments, inner and outer grief. It is the path of resolving suffering from the discrepancy between what you hoped for and the reality that was manifested. By the illuminating light of prayer and contemplation, many parts of you can be clarified and released of burdens, sorrows or regrets.

At a time like this, it is possible that the greatest pain is the pain of emptiness. This is a time to seek for, listen for and pray for wisdom and gratitude. It may feel as if the emptiness, pain and darkness will never end. As you bring more of your own spirit into the conversation with God, you may begin to find the light in the dark. You may see that out of the emptiness can come gratitude and wisdom. You may find that the act of releasing brings you to a new understanding. In this way, God can bring forth blessings out of darkness.

How can the darkness of this loss bring light to your soul? In the contemplative Christian tradition, it is believed that the greater the darkness encountered and the greater the contemplative search for meaning, the greater the purification of the soul. As this search for meaning preoccupies the soul and is focused intently on the absence of light and the absence of understanding, this search for meaning also propels you toward contemplation of the Divine. And to the extent that your will allows you to go in this direction, your soul seeks new meaning and understanding. It is believed that this seeking sheds new light. It is believed that the process of contemplation has the potential to affect the soul profoundly because in this process, the search for meaning moves the soul into the light of deep understanding and wisdom.

While working in the hospital, I met a 34 year old who was suffering from severe physical pain and emotional turmoil.

He had been shot multiple times late at night in a drug-infested neighborhood, and drugs may have played a role in his shooting. He almost died. He was at the hospital for several months and during that time he had undergone four critical operations to repair his leg, hip, foot and arm. The doctors expected him to lose the leg and be confined to a wheelchair for the rest of his life. Since he was confined to bed for many months, all he could think about was that his life was about to change dramatically for the worse. He told me he was terrified of losing his leg because he worked in construction and he would lose his livelihood. He was also expected to lose the use of one arm. He confessed his fear of living. He tossed and turned in pain. He wrestled with his soul for answers.

We met many times during the course of three months and he talked about his guilt, grief, anger, pain and fear. We prayed and offered this to God for healing. We did this over and over again. I encouraged him to seek the wisdom in the loss. He was baffled. He laughed at that idea and thought it was ridiculous. As time went by, he became more engaged in the prayers, and one day when I came by to see him, he was weeping in pain. He begged me to get more pain medication for him. I asked him if it was physical pain or emotional pain. He was unable to answer. He explained that he had been struggling with complicated feelings about his choices. He knew that he did not belong over there and that he should not have gone to that neighborhood in the middle of the night.

He talked about what he feared, what he regretted and what he wished he had done differently. He sobbed with regret for his circumstances, which he realized were the result of his own actions. I learned that he had been struggling to know God, and I invited him to express his grief. He wanted to know if God was listening; he wanted a "sign" that he was connected with God. We prayed that the sign would be the immediate end of the pain. By the time the prayer was over, he was asleep. The next day, he told me that his pain had completely disappeared during the prayer. He was thrilled and took this as a sign that God was there for him. His demeanor was radiant and his faith grew by leaps and bounds.

I left and continued on in my work, seeing other patients. About seven weeks later, he came by to see me. He was in a wheelchair, and he was eager to talk to me. I wondered what could be so urgent. Apparently, he had gone though this "dark night of the soul" and had emerged with newfound hope, excitement and vision for his future. The change in his outlook was startling. He told me that as a result of his near-death experience, he had made an emotional shift and found a new set of values.

He rejected his old beliefs about God (being boring, dull and uninspiring). He found a new worldview and new meaning.

He was growing emotionally. He was changing his personal affiliations, lifestyle, family priorities and his relationship to the Sacred.

During the dark and barren time suffering in the hospital, he had found an opportunity to open his heart, spirit and soul to Divine Love. He invited the Divine to enter his heart, and he was in the process of being transformed into a new person. He was glowing with joy and radiance. I could hardly believe my eyes. I realized in that moment he had found the courage to go on the journey to turn this tremendous loss to wisdom. He had sprung into a new energetic field filled with hope, joy and peace.

This is the journey you are invited to now.

Scripture Reading

You are invited to read the following scripture aloud:

"My soul weeps because of grief; strengthen me according to your word."

— Psalm 119:28

Contemplation

The goal of this last chapter is to help you find a sense of connection to the Sacred that is renewing, peaceful, moving, relevant and sublime. At this point, you are invited to explore how this loss has brought you to a new place of Acceptance, Gratitude, Peace, Understanding, Meaning, Purpose or Relationship to the Sacred. Please take some time to contemplate the following questions and write down your thoughts in the space provided:

1. What feelings and needs are you accepting now?
2. What could not have happened without this loss for which you are grateful?
3. What have you made **peace** with? (people, organizations or part of yourself)
4. What new **perspective** do you have now?
5. What new **understanding** has come from this loss?
6. What is the larger **meaning** of this loss for you?
7. How has this loss impacted your core **purpose**?
8. What is your relationship to the God and the **Sacred** as a result of this loss?

Write down your thoughts and feelings about acceptance, gratitude and peace. To what new realizations, understandings and ideas about your life's purpose you have come? How has your view of God changed?

_____
_____
_____
_____
_____
_____
_____
_____
_____
_____
_____
_____
_____
_____
_____
_____
_____
_____
_____
_____
_____

Please continue to the next page …

Candle-Lighting Prayer

It is my hope that as you complete the following Candle-Lighting Prayer, you will find glimmers of new understanding, new meaning and new purpose for your life. It is my hope that you will arrive at a place of acceptance and gratitude for what was given to you by the person or situation you lost. It is my further hope that you arrive at a sense of *peace* with yourself over the loss. And finally, I invite you to make room for the possibility that your relationship with God may have broadened, deepened or shifted in some way.

Recite these words aloud:

Welcome God
Wise and Gracious One
Lover of Goodness
Giver of Blessings
Creator of New Things,
Beloved Grace of Transformation and Renewal
Holder of Grief and Loss

I ask for Your blessed presence to oversee this prayer.
God of all history, God of all time, God of all futures,
Lead me. Show me the way forward in my life.
I confess the following feelings:

(Indicate what feelings you want to release and light a candle for each feeling. Say a few words about your current situation, including what you are leaving and what you are letting go of:)

_____

_____

_____

I ask for Your loving guidance to shepherd me forward.

God, help me envision the totality of Your grace and love.
God, surround me with Your Holy Spirit.
God, let me remember that I am made in Your image
God, thank you for Your goodness and grace in my life.
God, thank you for Your presence and blessings in my life.

Today, I release these burdens to You:
>   My anxiety, fear and hopelessness
>   My sorrow and grief
>   My anger and guilt
>   My loss and suffering

Gracious God, I ask that You take this grief, sorrow, loss and suffering.
Take the unceasing grief in my heart.
Move it through sorrow into wisdom.
Take my loss and suffering
Fill me with the warmth of Your loving heart.

Honor this waiting, despondent, empty time.

I lift up this empty time as time to cherish Your grace, abundance and love.
I lift up this despondent time as time to imagine and envision an abundant life.
I lift up the waiting time as time to imagine abundance in Your grace.

God, I ask Your blessing on this time
May I use it well
To reflect, pray and weep
To notice Your grace.

I invite the Holy Spirit to come forward,
To become my new foundation
And source of joy and abundance.

Welcome abundant Grace.
I open my heart to You this day.
I invite in Your abundance. (*Light candles to represent God's abundance.*)

Thank You God for Your abundant grace.

Movement toward Love

It is possible that you will not discover the blessings in your hardships until you have completely released blame, judgment, anger, resentment and guilt. That is why I recommend going back again to Chapter 1 to address the next strand of your grief and working it through each chapter. Work with each strand until every burden connected to your loss (situations, events, people, organizations) has been contemplated, prayed over and released to God.

As you complete your journey through this strand of loss, a sense of hopeful energy may begin to stir. The contemplative Christian tradition suggests that as soon as this emerges, a yearning arises for the Sacred to come forward. This can open the door for expanded love toward Self, others and God. This is the journey of the heart, spirit and soul through darkness ... into and out of despair, regret, shame, guilt, anger, blame and judgment.

It is believed that as the desire for God grows, spiritual longings become more important. This rotation of focus is filled with possibilities, especially the possibility of releasing old values while accepting new ones. This rotation creates space for the soul's thirst for love to be satisfied. The soul has a thirst for a love that honors truth, authentic emotional expression and creative expression of the heart's wisdom. You are invited to notice whatever shifts are taking place that might honor these possibilities and bring you into greater love of Self, others and God.

The release of grief can lead to a sense of mission and a reason for living, to new meaning and to a new way to view the world.

My hope is that you have found fresh understanding of your spiritual path, your connection with God and your inner growth journey as well as passion, understanding and hope.

Remember, suffering offers us a chance to connect with the Divine in new and authentic ways. Suffering can be a fruitful path for growth, wisdom and discernment. It can be a time when Spiritual Direction is welcome one can move out the old and embrace the new. It can be a time ripe for reconciliation.

And a time for miracles.

Final Blessing

Praise God
For this journey through loss and suffering
Praise God,
For Your courage and honesty
Praise God
For Blessings, Wisdom and new Understanding.

Glory to you, Glory to your journey and Glory be to God.

Resources

Co-Active Coaching, Laura Whitworth, Henry Kimsey-House and Phil Sandahl, Davies-Black Publishing, 1998.

Dark Night of the Soul, St. John of the Cross, translated and edited by E. Allison Peers, Doubleday, 1959.

Embracing Our Selves; the Voice Dialogue Manual, Hal and Sidra Stone, New World Library, 1989.

The Gift of Feeling, Paul Tournier, John Knox Press, 1979.

Giving Sorrow Words; Poems of Strength and Solace, Karren vanMeenen Editor, National Association of Poetry Therapy Foundation, 2002.

Guilt and Grace, Paul Tournier, Harper and Row Publishers, 1962.

HeartMath (www.hearthmath.org), a nonprofit research institute.

Lament for a Son, Nicholas Wollerstorff, William Eerdmans Publishing Co., 1987.

Opening our Hearts, Transforming our Losses, Al-Anon Family Group Headquarters, Inc., 2007.

The Power of Infinite Love and Gratitude, Dr. Darren Weissman, Hay House, 2005.

Prayers for Healing, 365 Blessings, Poems & Meditations from Around the World, Edited by Maggie Oman, Conari Press, 1999.

Psalms for Praying: An Invitation to Wholeness, Nan C. Merrill, Continuum Press, 2004.

Rachel's Cry, Prayer of Lament and Rebirth of Hope, Kathleen Billman & Daniel Migliore, United Church Press, 1999.

Rilke's Book of Hours, Love Poems to God, The Berkeley Publishing Group, Penguin, 2005.

Stages of Faith, The Psychology of Human Development and the Quest for Meaning, James W. Fowler, Harper Collins Publishers, 1981.

About The Author

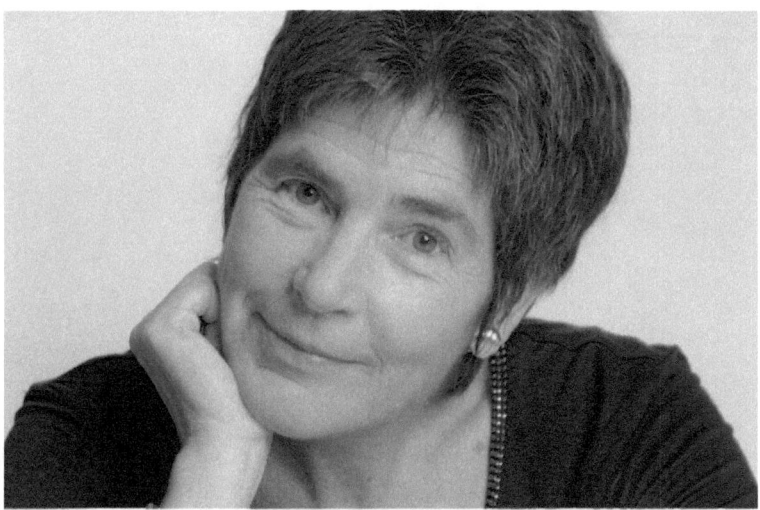

This book was created by Ms. Kramer to provide a guide to in-depth grieving with the goal of recovering and rebalancing completely. The foundation of this method is to dismantle the myth that grief lives with you forever. Ms. Kramer has worked with thousands of people who have followed this method successfully to process and release grief. She has proven that by focusing on the Divine, and seeking wisdom in the loss, it is possible to release grief and loss.

She uses a multidisciplinary approach that incorporates music, prayer, meditation, sone, movement and imagination. Through this approach, she has found that one can reorganize the way one sees and understands one's circumstances; and then reclaim direction, motivation and a sense of life's purpose.

Ms. Kramer has served as a hospital chaplain, grief counselor and hospice chaplain for UCSF Medical Center, Sutter Hospital and Heartland Hospice in Northern California. She received a Master of Arts degree in Public Health Administration, from the University of Michigan, a Master of Art's degree in Systematic Theology and a Master of Art's degree in Values from the Graduate Theological Union in Berkeley, California. She has also completed training programs and received certificates in Chaplaincy, Life Coaching and Spiritual Direction. Currently, she works as a Life Coach in the San Francisco bay area and may be reached through

www.kramercoaching.com

www.ingramcontent.com/pod-product-compliance
Lightning Source LLC
Chambersburg PA
CBHW020913080526
44589CB00011B/583